Intermittent Fasting For Men Over 60

A Complete Guide for Senior Men to Harness the Power of
Fasting, Boost Vitality, and Age with Strength

By

Olivia Stokes

Dear Reader,

Welcome to *INTERMITTENT FASTING FOR MEN OVER 60.*

I'm Olivia Stokes, a nutritionist deeply dedicated to helping individuals navigate the complexities of aging with vitality and resilience. With my extensive experience and unwavering commitment to promoting healthy living, I have crafted this comprehensive guide specifically designed to address the unique dietary and wellness needs of men over 60.

Recognizing the critical role that personalized nutrition and lifestyle choices play in maintaining health as we age, I am excited to share with you a range of delicious and nourishing recipes that will support your journey toward better health. Each recipe in this book has been thoughtfully chosen to align with the principles of intermittent fasting while also providing practical insights into managing health conditions commonly encountered in later life.

This book is a reflection of my passion and expertise, and I truly hope it empowers you to take charge of your health and well-being. As you explore these pages, I invite you to embrace this culinary journey, making positive changes and discovering new ways to fuel both your body and mind.

Your feedback is immensely valuable to me. It not only helps me improve as an author but also guides others on their health journeys. I encourage you to share your thoughts and experiences by leaving a review on Amazon. Your feedback will not only support my efforts but also assist others in making informed decisions about their well-being.

Thank you for choosing this book. Let's embark on this path together toward a healthier, more vibrant you.

Warm regards,

Olivia Stokes

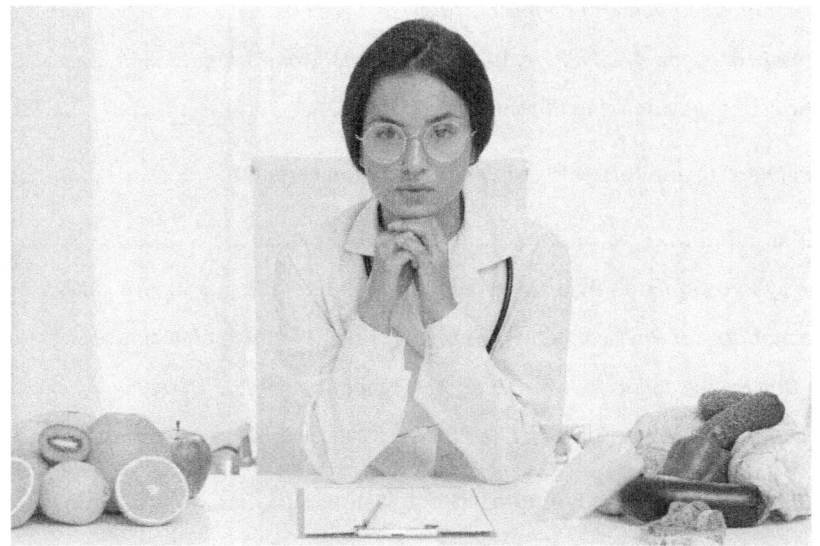

Table of Contents

Introduction...

Chapter 1: The Male Body After 60...10

1.1 Understanding Metabolic Changes in Men Over 60...10

1.2 The Decline of Human Growth Hormone (HGH) in Men Over 60...11

1.3 Additional Effects of Aging in Men Over 60..12

Chapter 2: Understanding Intermittent Fasting: A New Approach to Health for Men Over 60......14

2.1 Advantages of Intermittent Fasting for Men Over 60...15

2.2 Understanding the Realities of IF for Men Over 60..18

2.3 Risks of IF for Men Over 60 and How to Start Safely..19

2.3 Types of Intermittent Fasting..21

2.4 Combining Methods for Flexibility..28

2.5 Getting Started with Intermittent Fasting for Men Over 60..29

Chapter 3: Essential Foods for Men Over 60 Following IF..33

3.1 Recommended Foods for Intermittent Fasting...33

3.2 Suggested Food Items for Intermittent Fasting..34

3.3 Foods to Limit on an Intermittent Fasting Diet..36

3.4 Integrating Traditional Medicine and Natural Remedies with Intermittent Fasting for Men Over 60................36

3.5 Evaluating the Safety and Effectiveness of Supplements for Men Over 60...............................38

Chapter 4: Digital Health Tools and Trusted Resources for Men Over 60.....................................39

4.1 Reliable Websites..39

4.2 Online Communities and Support Forums...40

4.3 Recommended Academic Journals for Men Over 60...41

4.4 Digital Tools and Apps for Health and Wellness Monitoring..43

4.5 Resources for Managing Chronic Conditions...44

Chapter 5: Exercise and Intermittent Fasting for Men Over 60...46

....46

5.1 The Synergy of IFand Physical Activity for Men Over 60...46

5.2 Precautions for Physical Activity in Men Over 60 Practicing Intermittent Fasting.....................47

5.3 28-Day Exercise Plan for Men Over 60 (Compatible with IF Lifestyle).....................................49

5.4 Low-Impact Exercise for Men Over 60 Practicing Intermittent Fasting.....................................52

Chapter 6: Breakfast Recipes For Intermittent Fasting..54

1. Power Protein Smoothie..54

2. High-Protein Pancakes..54

3. Egg and Avocado on Sweet Potato Toast with Sautéed Kale..55

4. Sweet Potato and Turkey Breakfast Burritos..56

5. High-Fiber Banana Nut Porridge..57

6. Honey Almond Quinoa Granola..57

7. Savory Lentil & Veggie Scramble..58

8. Apple Cinnamon Almond Scones..59

9. Banana Walnut Oatmeal..60

10. Blueberry Almond Muffins..61

11. Egg Scramble with Sweet Potatoes..62

12. Sunflower Seed Butter Apple Toast..62

13. Egg and Cheese Quesadilla..63

14. Prune Walnut Energy Bites..64

15. Chickpea and Carrot Spread Sandwich..65

16. Cottage Cheese and Veggie Lettuce Wraps..65

17. Greek Yogurt with Apple and Almonds..66

18. Blueberry Spinach Smoothie..66

19. Quinoa Breakfast Bowl with Apple and Walnuts..67

20. Baked Pears with Almonds and Cinnamon..68

Chapter 6: Lunch Recipes For Intermittent Fasting..**70**

1. Lemon Herb Salmon with Roasted Brussels Sprouts..70

2. Grilled Eggplant and Spinach Panini..71

3. Sweet Potato and Black Bean Burrito..72

4. Lemon Herb Chicken and Veggie Skewers..73

5. Lemon Basil Grilled Cod..73

6. Lemon Garlic Shrimp Sauté..74

7. Butternut Squash and Spinach Risotto..75

8. Chickpea and Carrot Stew with Couscous..76

9. Chicken Salad with Walnuts and Grapes..77

10. Cauliflower Noodle Casserole..77

11. Mediterranean Shrimp Salad with Lemon Tahini Dressing..78

12. Zucchini Noodles with Spicy Peanut Sauce..79

13. Spicy Sweet Potato and Black Bean Quinoa Bowl..80

14. Greek-Style Chicken Salad Bowl..80

15. Bell Peppers Stuffed with Quinoa, Spinach, and Feta..81

16. Caper and Bean Salad with Tuna..82

17. Roasted Cauliflower and Broccoli Gratin..83

18. Spinach and Goat Cheese Omelette..83

19. Avocado and Kale Soup...84

20. Tropical Mango and Chicken Lettuce Wraps...85

Chapter 7: Dinner Recipes For Intermittent Fasting...**87**

1. Honey Sesame Salmon..87

2. Honey Garlic Tofu...88

3. Pork Tenderloin Stuffed with Apple, Walnuts, and Sage................................88

4. Roasted Carrots with Garlic and Herb Infusion...89

5. Herb-Crusted Baked Haddock..89

6. Citrus-Basil Baked Cod with Roasted Cherry Tomatoes................................90

7. Grilled Lemon Garlic Chicken Breasts...91

8. Maple-Balsamic Glazed Chicken Thighs with Roasted Butternut Squash....92

9. Citrus-Dijon Salmon with Roasted Cauliflower and Carrots.........................93

10. Herbed Chicken with Swiss Cheese...94

11. Ricotta and Sun-Dried Tomato Stuffed Salmon...94

12. Coconut Curried Pumpkin Soup..95

13. Eggplant Parmesan with Spinach and Avocado Salad...................................96

14. Lemon Rosemary Grilled Swordfish..97

15. Grilled Lamb Chops with Basil Pesto and Roasted Sweet Potatoes...........98

16. Sweet Potato and Rosemary Risotto...99

17. Herbed Spaghetti Squash with Roasted Bell Peppers and Feta................100

18. Walnut-Crusted Turkey Cutlets...100

19. Ginger-Lime Chicken with Cucumber and Bell Pepper Salad....................101

20. Stuffed Zucchini with Quinoa and Turkey..102

Chapter 8: Snack & Dessert Recipes For Intermittent Fasting..............................**103**

1. Coconut Chia Pudding with Mango..103

2. Peanut Butter Oatmeal Chocolate Chip Cookies...104

3. Spiced Almond-Coconut Energy Bites...104

4. Avocado-Cocoa Mousse with a Hint of Mint...105

5. Baked Pears with Cinnamon and Pecans...105

6. Carrot Oatmeal Raisin Muffins..106

7. Herbed Almonds with Rosemary...107

8. Chocolate Avocado Pudding...107

9. Berry Chia Seed Smoothie...108

10. Almond Butter Cookies..109

11. Creamy Coconut Rice Pudding with Chia Seeds..109

12. Coconut Carrot Crunch Cookies..110

13. Frozen Strawberry-Chocolate Greek Yogurt...111

14. Frozen Peach-Mint Greek Yogurt Bites..*111*

15. Cucumber Mint Raspberry Sorbet...*112*

16. Almond Butter and Apple Sushi Rolls...*112*

17. Nutty Oat Energy Bites...*113*

18. Mixed Berry Yogurt Parfait..*114*

90-Day Intermittent Fasting Meal Plan for Men Over 60..**115**

Conclusion..**126**

BONUS 1...**127**

BONUS ANTI-INFLAMMATORY RECIPES...**127**

BONUS 2...**128**

MUSIC FOR FASTING..**128**

Introduction

Entering the sixties can be a transformative experience for men—a time to reflect on life's accomplishments and consider how best to enjoy the years ahead. With this new chapter, many men find themselves focusing more on their health and well-being. However, the aging process can bring with it a series of physical changes that present challenges. Slower metabolism, increased difficulty in maintaining muscle mass, and weight gain are common issues men face after 60.

Despite these hurdles, there are effective ways to take control of one's health and vitality. Fasting on an intermittent basis (also known as IF) is one method that has garnered a lot of attention due to the fact that it has the ability to increase your general health. Fasting on an intermittent basis is not just another diet; rather, it is a way of life that can assist men in their sixties in managing their weight, improving their mental focus, and lowering their chance of developing chronic diseases.

For men over 60, changes in metabolism and hormonal balance can make it harder to maintain a healthy weight and muscle tone. Intermittent fasting can be a powerful tool to combat these changes. By alternating periods of eating with fasting, the body is encouraged to burn fat more efficiently, which can help men retain lean muscle and support metabolic health.

Beyond weight management, intermittent fasting offers a host of other health benefits that are particularly valuable for men in their sixties. Research shows that IF can help improve insulin sensitivity, which is key to avoiding type 2 diabetes—a common concern as men age. Additionally, intermittent fasting has been linked to reduced inflammation in the body, helping to lower the risk of heart disease and other chronic conditions that become more prevalent with age.

Intermittent fasting also supports cognitive health. According to a number of studies, fasting has the potential to improve brain function by stimulating the synthesis of brain-derived neurotrophic factor (BDNF), a protein that plays a role in the development and protection of brain cells. This can be crucial for maintaining mental clarity and memory as men move through their sixties, helping to ward off cognitive decline.

Choosing to incorporate intermittent fasting into daily life can be a transformative step towards healthier aging. It empowers men over 60 to embrace this stage of life with renewed strength, mental acuity, and vitality. With the right approach, intermittent fasting can help men live their sixties with confidence, energy, and a proactive approach to longevity.

Chapter 1: The Male Body After 60

1.1 Understanding Metabolic Changes in Men Over 60

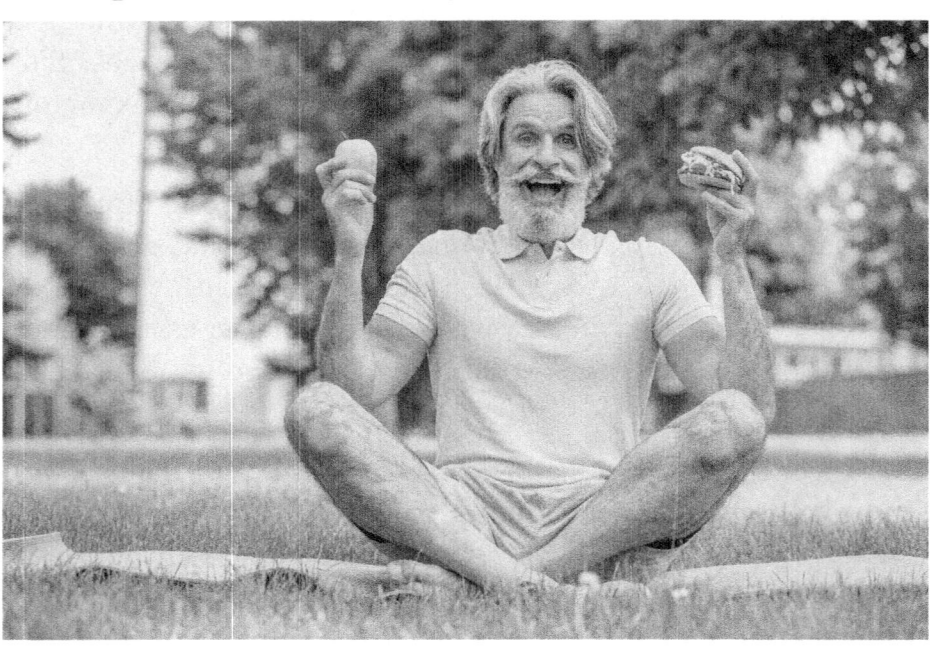

As men enter their sixties, they often notice changes in their bodies that were not present in earlier years. One of the most significant shifts occurs in the body's metabolism. The process by which the body turns sustenance and liquids into usable energy is referred to as metabolism. As men age, this process naturally begins to slow down, leading to a variety of effects, including weight gain and a reduction in overall energy levels. For men over 60, this slowing metabolism can be particularly frustrating. Even if they maintain the same eating habits and activity levels as they did in their younger years, many men find it more difficult to manage their weight. This is because, as metabolism slows, the body burns fewer calories at rest. Simply put, the energy expenditure that used to come naturally now requires more conscious effort.

One major factor influencing metabolic rate in older men is the decrease in muscle mass that typically accompanies aging. When opposed to adipose tissue, muscle tissue is metabolically active, which means that it takes a greater amount of energy to be maintained. Men have a tendency to experience a loss of muscle mass as they age, a condition known as sarcopenia, which is a factor that leads to a slower metabolism. This loss of muscle mass makes it more challenging to stay lean and can also lead to a decrease in strength and mobility.

In addition to sarcopenia, hormonal changes play a critical role in metabolic shifts for men over 60. Men see a gradual decrease in testosterone levels as they age. Testosterone is the hormone that is important to preserve bone density, muscle mass, and sex desire. This drop in testosterone levels is a significant contributor to the changes in body composition that many men experience. Lower testosterone can result in increased fat storage, particularly around the abdomen, and a reduction in lean muscle mass. These changes not only affect appearance but also impact overall metabolic health.

The interaction between metabolism and hormones creates a feedback loop that can exacerbate weight gain and muscle loss. As metabolism slows, it becomes easier to gain weight, and the more weight a man gains, particularly in the form of fat, the more it can negatively impact hormone levels. For example, excess fat tissue can lead to higher levels of estrogen, a hormone that can further reduce testosterone levels in men, creating a cycle that makes it even more difficult to lose weight and maintain muscle mass.

Another important factor to consider is insulin sensitivity. This is because as men become older, their cells may become less receptive to insulin, which is the hormone that controls the amount of sugar in their blood. This disease, which is referred to as insulin resistance, can result in elevated levels of blood sugar as well as an increased likelihood of getting type 2 diabetes. Insulin resistance is closely linked to metabolic health and is often exacerbated by weight gain, especially around the abdomen.

Maintaining a healthy metabolism after 60 requires a combination of strategies, including regular physical activity, a balanced diet, and potentially, intermittent fasting. Exercise, particularly strength training, is crucial for preserving muscle mass and supporting metabolic health. In addition to its physical benefits, exercise can help regulate hormone levels, improving testosterone production and overall metabolic function.

Dietary habits also play a significant role in managing metabolism as men age. Consuming nutrient-dense foods that are rich in protein can support muscle maintenance, while minimizing processed foods and sugar can help manage weight and reduce the risk of insulin resistance. Intermittent fasting, in particular, has shown promise as a method for improving metabolic health by allowing the body to reset its insulin sensitivity and promote fat loss while preserving lean muscle.

While aging inevitably brings about changes in metabolism, it is possible to manage and even mitigate some of these effects through lifestyle choices. By understanding the unique challenges that come with aging and implementing targeted strategies, men over 60 can maintain a healthy metabolism, supporting their overall well-being and quality of life.

1.2 The Decline of Human Growth Hormone (HGH) in Men Over 60

As men age, one of the key hormonal changes they experience is the gradual decline in the production of HGH. HGH is an essential hormone that is generated by the pituitary gland. It is associated with growth, the regeneration of cells, and the maintenance of healthy tissues throughout an individual's lifetime. In youth, HGH levels are high, supporting muscle growth, fat metabolism, and overall vitality. However, as men enter their 60s, HGH production decreases significantly, leading to noticeable changes in the body. The decline in HGH is often linked to some of the most common challenges faced by men over 60, such as the loss of muscle mass, an increase in body fat, particularly around the abdomen, and reduced energy levels. HGH is essential for maintaining muscle tissue, and as its levels drop, so does the body's ability to repair and build muscle. This can lead to sarcopenia, the age-related loss of muscle mass, which not only affects strength and mobility but also contributes to a slower metabolism.

HGH is essential for the metabolism of fat and its involvement in the maintenance of muscle. It is easier for the body to convert fat into energy when the levels of HGH are high. However, as HGH declines, fat metabolism slows down, making it easier for men to gain weight, especially in the form of visceral fat around the abdomen. Because it is linked to an increased risk of cardiovascular disease, diabetes, and other metabolic problems, this specific kind of fat is very hazardous to one's health. The decrease in HGH also impacts overall vitality and recovery. Men over 60 may find that they no longer recover as quickly from physical activity or injuries, and their energy levels may not be what they once were. This is because HGH plays a critical role in cell regeneration and repair. When levels are lower, the body's ability to repair itself is diminished, leading to longer recovery times and a general feeling of fatigue. Furthermore, HGH has a strong influence on skin health and elasticity. As HGH levels decrease, men may notice that their skin becomes thinner, less elastic, and more prone to wrinkles. While this is a natural part of aging, the decline in HGH accelerates these visible signs of aging. Given the significant impact of HGH on various aspects of health, many men over 60 are interested in ways to support or even boost their natural HGH levels. One approach that has shown promise is intermittent fasting. Studies suggest that intermittent fasting can stimulate the body's production of HGH. When the body is in a fasted state, HGH levels can increase, helping to preserve muscle mass and promote fat burning, even as overall production of the hormone decreases with age. This makes intermittent fasting a potentially valuable tool for older men looking to counteract some of the effects of HGH decline.

In addition to intermittent fasting, regular exercise, particularly strength training, can also support HGH production. Exercise stimulates the release of HGH, especially during high-intensity workouts. Strength training, in particular, is effective at preserving muscle mass and boosting metabolism, making it a crucial component of a healthy lifestyle for men over 60.

Adequate sleep is another important factor in maintaining healthy HGH levels. The majority of HGH is released during deep sleep, particularly during the first few hours of the night. In light of this, ensuring proper sleep hygiene and striving for seven to nine hours of quality sleep each night can assist in optimizing the body's natural generation of HGH.

1.3 Additional Effects of Aging in Men Over 60

Aging brings about numerous changes in the male body, and while some of these changes are expected, they can still be challenging to navigate. Beyond the slowing metabolism and the decline in HGH production, men over 60 face other significant physiological and psychological shifts that impact their overall health and quality of life. Understanding these changes and taking proactive steps to manage them is crucial for maintaining vitality and well-being during this stage of life. One of the most significant hormonal changes men experience after 60 is the gradual decline in testosterone levels, a phenomenon sometimes referred to as andropause or male menopause. Testosterone is the hormone responsible for regulating a wide range of functions in the male body, including maintaining muscle mass, bone density, and sexual health. As men become older, their testosterone levels naturally start to decrease, which can result in a variety of signs and symptoms, both physically and emotionally. A decline in testosterone can result in reduced muscle mass and strength, contributing to the challenges of sarcopenia.

This loss of muscle might make it more difficult for men to maintain an active lifestyle, which in turn can improve their risk of falling and becoming injured. A low testosterone level is associated with lower bone density, which in turn raises the risk of osteoporosis and fractures. This is in spite of the impact that it has on muscles. This is why strength training and weight-bearing exercises are often recommended for older men to help maintain both muscle and bone health.

Another consequence of lower testosterone levels is a reduction in libido and sexual function. Many men over 60 experience changes in their sexual health, including erectile dysfunction and a decrease in overall sexual desire. While these changes are normal, they can sometimes affect a man's self-esteem and relationships. It's important for men to be aware that there are various treatment options available, and discussing concerns with a healthcare provider can help in managing these issues effectively.

In addition to hormonal shifts, the aging process also brings an increased focus on prostate health. The disease known as BPH is characterized by an increase in the size of the prostate gland as a result of aging. This enlargement can cause urinary issues, such as increased frequency, urgency, and difficulty in starting urination. While BPH is not typically life-threatening, it can significantly impact a man's quality of life. Monitoring the health of the prostate and addressing any possible problems at an earlier stage can be accomplished through routine checkups with a healthcare provider. Moreover, maintaining a healthy diet, staying active, and managing stress can all contribute to better prostate health as men age.

Cardiovascular health is another area of concern for men over 60. The loss of flexibility in the blood arteries and the increased effort required by the heart to pump blood throughout the body are two of the factors that contribute to an increased risk of cardiovascular disease, hypertension, and stroke as one ages. Factors such as high cholesterol, high blood pressure, and lifestyle habits like smoking and poor diet can further exacerbate these risks. Incorporating regular physical activity, particularly cardiovascular exercise, along with a diet rich in heart-healthy foods, can help men protect their heart health as they age. Furthermore, it has been demonstrated that intermittent fasting has positive benefits on the health of the heart by lowering levels of inflammation, enhancing cholesterol levels, and promoting healthy blood pressure.

Mental health is another critical aspect of aging that should not be overlooked. Men over 60 may be more susceptible to depression, anxiety, and feelings of isolation, particularly as they transition into retirement, experience the loss of loved ones, or face health challenges. The stigma around mental health in men can sometimes prevent them from seeking help, leading to untreated symptoms that can affect their overall well-being. It is of the utmost importance to acknowledge that mental health is equally vital as physical health and to seek support that is available online, whether through therapy, support groups, or loved ones, can make a significant difference. It may be possible to lessen the impact of these consequences by including behaviors that are beneficial to mental health, such as practicing mindfulness, engaging in regular physical activity, and keeping up social connections. There is some evidence that intermittent fasting can have a beneficial effect on mental health by enhancing brain health and lowering inflammatory levels, which has been linked to mood disorders.

Chapter 2: Understanding Intermittent Fasting: A New Approach to Health for Men Over 60

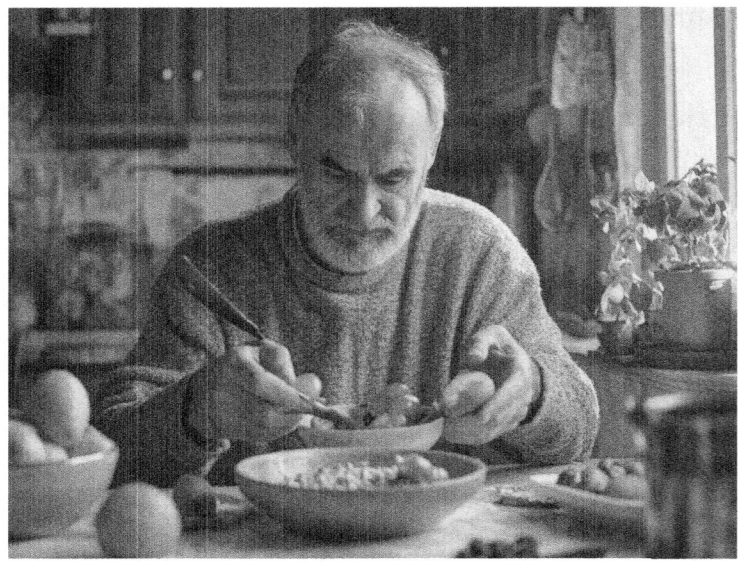

The practice of intermittent fasting is currently experiencing a boom in popularity, particularly as a remedy for enhancing one's health and controlling one's weight. However, the practice of fasting is far from new. Throughout history, many cultures have embraced fasting not only for religious or spiritual reasons but also as a means to enhance physical performance and mental clarity. For instance, ancient warriors and athletes, including those from the Greek and Roman civilizations, often fasted to prepare their bodies for battle or competition. So, what is intermittent fasting, and how does it stand apart from traditional fasting? More importantly, can following specific eating windows truly contribute to weight loss and better health, particularly for men over 60?

IF, which stands for intermittent fasting, is not a diet in the traditional sense; rather, it is a pattern of eating that varies between intervals of eating and periods of fasting alternating with one another. In contrast to many diets, which place an emphasis on restricting particular foods or monitoring calories, intermittent fasting places more emphasis on the timing of meals instead of the foods themselves. This makes it an appealing option for men who prefer flexibility in their food choices while still seeking significant health benefits. One of the key reasons intermittent fasting has gained traction is its positive impact on metabolic health. For men over 60, this can be especially valuable. As metabolism naturally slows with age, maintaining a healthy weight and preventing metabolic disorders become more challenging. IF helps by lowering insulin levels, which allows the body to burn fat more efficiently and stabilize energy levels throughout the day.

There are various approaches to intermittent fasting, all of which involve structured periods of eating followed by periods of fasting. You might choose to eat only during specific hours each day, or follow a schedule where you fast for entire days at regular intervals during the week. The key is consistency, as this allows your body to adapt to the fasting pattern. Unlike other diet plans, intermittent fasting doesn't require strict food rules or tedious meal planning. Instead, it seamlessly integrates into your existing routine, making it more of a lifestyle shift than a temporary fix. In addition to promoting weight loss, intermittent fasting may also have a number of other possible health benefits for males over the age of 60.

It can help lower the risk of diabetes and heart disease, two of the most common health concerns as men age. Additionally, it has been shown to preserve muscle mass, which is crucial for maintaining strength and mobility. Cognitive benefits are also significant, with fasting promoting better mental clarity and potentially lowering the risk of neurodegenerative diseases. One of the major advantages of intermittent fasting is its simplicity. By reducing the number of meals you prepare and eat each day, it streamlines meal planning and cuts down on time spent in the kitchen. This makes it a practical and sustainable approach for older men who may be looking for ways to improve their health without overhauling their entire lifestyle. We have already touched on several key benefits of intermittent fasting, including improved metabolic health, better cardiovascular function, and enhanced hormone balance. In the following sections, we will delve deeper into these advantages, exploring in greater detail how intermittent fasting can specifically address the health challenges faced by men over 60 and contribute to overall well-being.

2.1 Advantages of Intermittent Fasting for Men Over 60

As men enter their 60s, the challenges of aging become more prominent, and maintaining optimal health requires a proactive approach. One powerful tool that has gained substantial attention for its wide-ranging health benefits is intermittent fasting (IF). While the concept of intermittent fasting may initially seem daunting, its flexibility and scientific backing make it a suitable lifestyle choice for men over 60 who are looking to progress their health, longevity, and overall quality of life. Intermittent fasting offers a range of benefits that are particularly valuable for older men. These benefits extend beyond simple weight management, influencing key areas such as metabolic health, cardiovascular function, testosterone levels, prostate health, and even the prevention of age-related diseases.

Weight Management and Fat Loss. The ability of intermittent fasting to effectively regulate weight is one of the most well-known advantages of this weight loss method. As men get older, their metabolism automatically slows down, which makes it more difficult for them to keep their weight at a healthy level. In males over the age of sixty, the buildup of visceral fat, especially in the abdominal region, can cause a rise in the likelihood of a number of different health issues, including diabetes and cardiovascular disease. Intermittent fasting helps men manage their weight by creating structured periods of calorie restriction, which in turn leads to fat loss without the need for strict diets or calorie counting. A further benefit of intermittent fasting is that it has been demonstrated to facilitate fat loss while simultaneously keeping lean muscular mass. This is particularly important for older men, as maintaining muscle becomes increasingly difficult with age. By preserving muscle mass and promoting fat burning, intermittent fasting offers a balanced approach to weight management that supports both physical health and functional mobility.

Enhanced Metabolic Health. Due to the fact that the risk of developing disorders such as insulin resistance, type 2 diabetes, and metabolic syndrome increases with age, men over the age of 60 should be extremely concerned about their metabolic health. Through the enhancement of insulin sensitivity and the reduction of blood sugar levels, intermittent fasting has a significant impact on the improvement of metabolically healthy individuals. For older men, this means a lower risk of developing diabetes and other metabolic disorders that can significantly impair quality of life.

Research shows that intermittent fasting can reduce fasting insulin levels by 20-30%, making it a powerful tool for managing blood sugar. This improvement in insulin sensitivity also helps in reducing chronic inflammation, which is linked to numerous age-related diseases, including cardiovascular disease and certain cancers. By incorporating intermittent fasting into their routine, men over 60 can better manage their metabolic health, reducing the risk of serious health complications.

Cardiovascular Benefits. Cardiovascular disease remains one of the leading causes of death among men over 60. As men age, the risk of developing heart conditions, such as high blood pressure, atherosclerosis, and heart attacks, increases significantly. Intermittent fasting has been shown to have several positive effects on cardiovascular health, making it a valuable practice for men who are concerned about heart disease. The practice of intermittent fasting has been shown to decrease levels of LDL cholesterol, lower blood pressure, and enhance the overall function of the heart. Furthermore, fasting encourages autophagy, which is a biological mechanism that assists in the removal of damaged cells and brings about a reduction in the accumulation of dangerous plaques in the arteries. This process can help lower the risk of heart attacks and strokes, making intermittent fasting a heart-healthy choice for men in their golden years.

Testosterone and Hormonal Balance. The possible impact that intermittent fasting may have on testosterone levels and hormonal balance is one of the advantages of this practice that is less well-known for men over the age of 60. Testosterone plays a vital role in men's health, influencing everything from muscle mass and strength to libido and energy levels. Unfortunately, as people become older, their testosterone levels gradually decrease, which can result in symptoms such as weariness, decreased sexual drive, and loss of muscle. Through the promotion of fat loss and the improvement of insulin sensitivity, intermittent fasting has been demonstrated to improve testosterone levels and support healthy living. Due to the fact that fat cells have the ability to convert testosterone into estrogen, having an excessive amount of body fat, particularly visceral fat, could lead to reduced testosterone levels. By reducing body fat through intermittent fasting, men may experience an improvement in their testosterone levels, leading to enhanced energy, vitality, and overall well-being. Moreover, intermittent fasting has been linked to increased human growth hormone (HGH) production, which works synergistically with testosterone to preserve muscle mass, support fat burning, and promote recovery. This hormonal boost is especially beneficial for men over 60 who want to maintain their physical performance and quality of life as they age.

Prostate Health and Cancer Prevention. The health of the prostate is a key issue for men over the age of 60, as disorders such as BPH and prostate cancer progressively grow more common with increasing age. Intermittent fasting may offer protective benefits for the prostate by reducing inflammation and supporting cellular repair through autophagy. By promoting healthier cellular function, intermittent fasting can potentially lower the risk of prostate-related issues. Furthermore, there is a possibility that intermittent fasting could have a role in the prevention of cancer by enhancing the body's capacity to repair DNA and lowering oxidative stress simultaneously, both of which are critical factors in cancer development.

While more research is needed specifically on prostate cancer and intermittent fasting, the general anti-inflammatory and autophagic benefits of fasting suggest that it could be a helpful practice for reducing cancer risk in older men.

Cognitive Health and Mental Clarity. As men get older, maintaining their mental health and cognitive function becomes equally vital. Research has shown that intermittent fasting can provide cognitive benefits that are beneficial to maintain brain health. In the brain, the process of fasting stimulates the creation of a protein known as BDNF, which is responsible for promoting the growth and survival of neurons. This has the potential to provide protection against neurodegenerative disorders such as Parkinson's and Alzheimer's, both of which are more prevalent in people who are in their later years. In addition to its neuroprotective effects, intermittent fasting may also improve mental clarity and focus. Many people report feeling more mentally sharp and energized during fasting periods, which can be particularly beneficial for older men who want to stay mentally active and engaged.

Improved Joint Health and Mobility. As men age, joint health can deteriorate, leading to conditions such as arthritis and decreased mobility. Intermittent fasting has been linked to decreased inflammation and improved joint health. By lowering overall inflammation in the body, fasting can help alleviate joint pain and stiffness, promoting better mobility and physical comfort.

Enhanced Longevity. Research that is only beginning to emerge indicates that intermittent fasting might have a role in improving healthier longevity. Studies have shown that fasting can activate cellular repair processes and enhance the body's resilience to age-related diseases. By adopting intermittent fasting, men over 60 might not only improve their current health but also potentially extend their lifespan.

Digestive Health: Digestive issues such as bloating, constipation, and indigestion are common concerns for older adults. Intermittent fasting can contribute to improved digestive health by giving the gut a regular rest period, which may enhance digestion and nutrient absorption. The structured eating periods can help regulate bowel movements and reduce discomfort.

Improved Sleep Quality. Quality sleep often declines with age, affecting overall health and well-being. Intermittent fasting can positively influence sleep patterns by stabilizing blood sugar levels and reducing late-night eating, which is known to disrupt sleep. Improved sleep can contribute to better mood, energy levels, and cognitive function.

Reduced Risk of Frailty. Frailty is a common condition in older adults characterized by weakness, weight loss, and reduced physical activity. Intermittent fasting, by promoting muscle preservation and reducing fat, can help mitigate the risk of frailty. Maintaining a healthy weight and muscle mass through fasting can support physical strength and independence.

Mental Resilience and Stress Management. The structured nature of intermittent fasting can enhance mental resilience by providing a sense of routine and control. This can help men manage stress better and improve overall emotional well-being. Additionally, the mental clarity often reported during fasting periods can contribute to a more positive outlook and better stress management.

Improved Skin Health. Aging skin can become thinner and less elastic, leading to wrinkles and dryness. Intermittent fasting may support skin health by reducing oxidative stress and promoting cellular repair processes. This can contribute to healthier, more resilient skin.

2.2 Understanding the Realities of IF for Men Over 60

Intermittent fasting (IF) has garnered attention as a promising strategy for improving health and managing weight, especially for men over 60. While it offers numerous benefits, it's essential to understand what intermittent fasting truly entails and how it fits into a broader health strategy. Here's a closer look at the realities of intermittent fasting, its effectiveness, and considerations for those in their later years.

Intermittent Fasting: More Than Just a Weight Loss Tool

Intermittent fasting is often touted as an effective weight management approach, but it's important to recognize that it may not always be faster or more effective than other methods of calorie control. While IF can enhance metabolic activity and contribute to overall health, it operates differently than traditional daily calorie restriction. As part of the practice of intermittent fasting, one alternates between times of eating and fasting, which can offer unique health benefits beyond simple weight loss. For men over 60, incorporating intermittent fasting can be particularly beneficial due to its potential impact on metabolism, hormone levels, and overall health. However, the effectiveness of IF in achieving rapid weight loss compared to continuous calorie restriction is still a subject of ongoing research. What is clear is that intermittent fasting can lead to significant health improvements when paired with a balanced and nutritious diet. To maximize the gains of intermittent fasting, it is crucial to focus on what you eat during the eating windows. Simply adhering to a fasting schedule without considering the quality of your diet can undermine the positive effects of fasting. Consuming high-calorie, nutrient-poor foods during non-fasting periods can counteract the benefits of intermittent fasting and potentially lead to weight gain or nutritional deficiencies. A diet that is abundant in whole foods, lean proteins, healthy fats, and a large quantity of fruits and vegetables is the ideal diet for men over the age of 60. This balanced approach helps ensure that the body receives the necessary nutrients for preserving muscle mass, supporting metabolic health, and enhancing general health. Adjusting to intermittent fasting can be challenging, particularly during the initial phase when the body is adapting to longer periods without food. It's common to experience hunger or discomfort as you transition to a new eating pattern, such as skipping breakfast. However, persistence can lead to improved adaptation and a smoother fasting experience. For those who find the adjustment period difficult, drinking beverages like black coffee or green tea during fasting hours can help manage hunger without significantly impacting insulin levels. These options can extend the fasting period and alleviate some of the initial discomfort associated with fasting.

It is essential to acknowledge that intermittent fasting is not a quick fix but instead a lifestyle choice that may be maintained over time and can be used in conjunction with a more comprehensive and comprehensive health strategy. It can be especially advantageous for men over 60 who are looking to maintain their health while adapting their eating habits.

However, the approach may not be suitable for everyone, particularly those who experience adverse symptoms such as severe cravings, migraines, or low blood sugar levels. Consultation with a qualified medical practitioner is very necessary prior to beginning intermittent fasting, particularly if you already have preexisting health concerns or specific dietary requirements from the beginning. Men over 60 should seek guidance from their primary care physician and, if possible, a registered dietitian. This ensures that intermittent fasting aligns with their individual health goals and conditions. As dietary trends evolve, intermittent fasting continues to gain popularity due to its potential health benefits and flexible approach. However, it's important to approach it with a balanced perspective, considering both its advantages and potential limitations. Ongoing research and personal experimentation will further clarify its role in maintaining health and well-being in older adults.

2.3 Risks of IF for Men Over 60 and How to Start Safely

Intermittent fasting (IF) can offer numerous benefits, particularly for men over 60, such as improved weight management, better metabolic health, and enhanced energy levels. Nevertheless, it is of the utmost importance to be made aware of the potential dangers that are involved with intermittent fasting, especially in older adults. This section will explore the risks and provide strategies for safely integrating intermittent fasting into your lifestyle.

Potential Risks of Intermittent Fasting for Men Over 60

1. Nutrient Deficiencies. As men age, maintaining adequate nutrient intake becomes increasingly important due to changes in digestion and absorption. In the absence of proper management, intermittent fasting can occasionally result in deficits in certain nutrients. When the eating window is restricted, there is a possibility that the individual will not consume enough of the vital vitamins and minerals that are necessary for maintaining overall health and an extended lifespan. There is a possibility that you are deficient in certain essential nutrients, such as vitamin D, calcium, and B vitamins. These nutrients are essential for maintaining healthy bones, producing energy, and functioning cognitively.

2. Blood Sugar Fluctuations. Intermittent fasting can cause fluctuations in blood sugar levels, which may be particularly concerning for men with diabetes or other blood sugar disorders. The periods of fasting can lead to hypoglycemia (low blood sugar) or hyperglycemia (high blood sugar), based on the individual's response and medication regimen. Proper management is crucial to prevent complications, such as dizziness, fatigue, and even more severe health issues.

3. Muscle Loss. Preserving muscle mass is essential for maintaining functional strength and mobility in older adults. Prolonged fasting or extreme calorie restriction can contribute to muscle loss, especially if protein intake is insufficient. This can be a concern for men over 60 who are already at risk of sarcopenia (age-related muscle loss). Muscle maintenance requires a balanced diet rich in protein and regular resistance training, which may be challenged by some intermittent fasting regimens.

4. Dehydration. During fasting periods, especially in the early stages, men may be at risk of dehydration. Fasting can reduce fluid intake inadvertently, leading to dehydration, particularly if not enough water is consumed. Symptoms of dehydration include dry mouth, dark urine, and fatigue. For older adults, dehydration can exacerbate existing health conditions and lead to complications such as kidney stones or urinary tract infections.

5. Electrolyte Imbalances. Extended fasting can lead to imbalances in electrolytes, such as sodium, potassium, and magnesium. These imbalances can affect heart health and overall bodily functions. Older adults, in particular, may have a reduced ability to regulate electrolyte levels due to age-related changes in kidney function and overall health.

6. Increased Risk of Gallstones. For some individuals, fasting can lead to an increased risk of gallstones, especially if fasting periods are prolonged or if there is a significant weight loss. Gallstones can cause pain and digestive issues and may require medical intervention.

Strategies for Safe Intermittent Fasting for Men Over 60

- **Start Gradually.** When beginning intermittent fasting for the first time, it is best to begin slowly so that your body has time to adjust to the new routine. Start out with fasting for shorter periods of time, such as twelve hours, and slowly boost the length of time you fast as you feel more at ease with the practice. This approach helps minimize potential side effects and makes the transition smoother.

- **Consult Healthcare Professionals.** Before beginning any kind of fasting routine, it is essential to discuss the matter with your healthcare professional, as was indicated earlier. This is especially important if you have any pre-existing problems, such as diabetes, hypertension, or cardiovascular concerns. The transition to intermittent fasting can be made easier with the assistance of a healthcare practitioner who can provide individualized guidance and monitor your health conditions.

- **Focus on Balanced Nutrition.** When you are eating, be sure that you are consuming a diet that is both well-balanced and abundant in the nutrients that your body needs. For the purpose of satisfying your nutritional requirements, you should consume a wide range of fruits, vegetables, whole grains, lean proteins, and healthy fats. Pay attention to protein intake to support muscle maintenance and overall health. Deficiencies can be avoided and your general health can be supported by consuming meals that are rich in nutrients.

- **Stay Hydrated.** Consuming the appropriate amount of water is essential, especially during periods of fasting. Be sure to consume a lot of water throughout the day, and if necessary, you should also think about include electrolyte-rich beverages in your diet. Because they might contribute to dehydration, coffee and alcohol should be avoided in excessive amounts. Urine that is light in color is normally indicative of appropriate hydration, whereas urine that is dark in color may be indicative of dehydration. Monitoring the color of urine can be a simple approach to determine the amount of hydration.

- **Monitor Blood Sugar Levels.** If you have diabetes or other blood sugar-related conditions, regularly monitor your blood sugar levels to ensure they remain stable. Adjust your fasting and eating plans based on your glucose readings and any advice provided by your healthcare provider. Be mindful of symptoms like dizziness or weakness, which could indicate blood sugar imbalances.

- **Incorporate Regular Physical Activity.** Blend intermittent fasting with a balanced exercise routine to support muscle maintenance and overall health. Engage in regular physical activity, including resistance training and aerobic exercises, to counteract muscle loss and support cardiovascular health. Exercise can also help manage stress and improve overall energy levels.

- **Listen to Your Body.** When you are fasting intermittently, pay attention to how your body reacts to the change. If you are experiencing substantial discomfort, exhaustion, or other undesirable symptoms, you should think about changing your fasting schedule or contacting with a healthcare specialist. When it comes to maintaining your general health and well-being, it is absolutely necessary to pay attention to your body and make adjustments as needed.

- **Plan Meals Wisely.** Ensure that your meals during eating windows are nutrient-rich and well-balanced. Planning ahead can help you make healthier choices and avoid the temptation of high-calorie or processed foods. The act of preparing meals in advance can not only save time but also make it simpler to adhere to a set of healthy eating guidelines.

- **Address Digestive Health.** If you experience digestive issues like bloating or constipation, focus on incorporating fiber-rich foods and staying hydrated. Fiber helps regulate digestion and can alleviate some common digestive problems associated with fasting.

In summary, while intermittent fasting can offer valuable health benefits for men over 60, it is crucial to be aware of and manage potential risks. By starting gradually, consulting with healthcare professionals, maintaining balanced nutrition, and listening to your body, you can safely integrate intermittent fasting into your lifestyle and enjoy its benefits.

2.3 Types of Intermittent Fasting

Intermittent fasting (IF) encompasses a variety of approaches, each with its own set of advantages and challenges. For men over 60, selecting the right intermittent fasting method can be crucial for achieving health goals while minimizing potential risks. This chapter provides a comprehensive overview of the most popular types of intermittent fasting, their benefits, and their considerations for older men.

1. THE 16/8 METHOD

The 16/8 approach, which is often referred to as time-restricted eating, is abstaining from food for a period of sixteen hours and then eating during a window of eight hours each day. For instance, one might eat between 10 a.m. and 6 p.m., fasting from 6 p.m. until 10 a.m. the next day.

Benefits for Men Over 60

- **Weight Management:** Because of this strategy, general calorie consumption can be reduced, which in turn encourages fat loss, which can be beneficial for men struggling with age-related weight gain.

- **Improved Metabolic Health:** By allowing the body to fast for extended periods, insulin sensitivity improves, which can lower the risk of type 2 diabetes.

- **Simplified Eating Schedule:** The 16/8 method is relatively easy to integrate into daily life without complex meal planning or drastic dietary changes.

Drawbacks for Men Over 60

- **Initial Adjustment Period:** Older men may experience hunger or irritability when initially adjusting to a 16-hour fasting period.

- **Potential for Nutrient Deficiency:** If not carefully managed, the restricted eating window might lead to inadequate nutrient intake, particularly important for maintaining bone health and muscle mass.

Strategy for Success

- **Gradual Transition:** Begin with a shorter time of fasting, such as 12 hours, and slowly raise it to 16 hours every day from there.

- **Focus on Nutrient-Dense Foods:** Ensure that meals within the 8-hour window are balanced and rich in essential nutrients to meet dietary needs.

2. THE 5:2 METHOD

The 5:2 technique is eating regularly for five days of the week and then dramatically decreasing the amount of calories consumed on two days that are not consecutive, often with the goal of consuming between 500 and 600 calories each day.

Benefits for Men Over 60

- **Flexible Approach:** The 5:2 method allows for normal eating on most days, which can be less restrictive and easier to maintain long-term.

- **Reduced Risk of Chronic Diseases:** Research suggests that periodic calorie restriction can aid in decreasing the danger of cardiovascular diseases and improve metabolic markers.

- **Potential for Improved Longevity:** The 5:2 method has been associated with benefits related to aging and longevity, which is appealing for older men.

Drawbacks for Men Over 60

- **Potential Fatigue:** On fasting days, calorie restriction may lead to low energy levels, which can be challenging for older men, especially those with existing health issues.

- **Nutritional Balance:** Maintaining a balanced diet on non-fasting days is crucial to avoid nutrient deficiencies, which can be more challenging as metabolic rates change with age.

Strategy for Success

- **Choose Low-Calorie, Nutrient-Rich Foods:** On fasting days, focus on high-fiber and high-protein foods to stay satiated.

- **Stay Hydrated:** Drink plenty of water and herbal teas to manage hunger and maintain hydration.

3. ALTERNATE-DAY FASTING (ADF)

By switching between days of normal eating and days of complete or near-complete fasting, the Alternate-Day Fasting method allows one to achieve a healthier lifestyle. On fasting days, some variants allow for minimal calorie intake (about 500 calories).

Benefits for Men Over 60

- **Enhanced Metabolic Health:** This method can significantly improve insulin sensitivity and aid in weight loss.

- **Potential for Significant Fat Loss:** The alternating fasting approach can lead to considerable fat loss, which may be beneficial for managing age-related fat accumulation.

Drawbacks for Men Over 60

- **Difficulty with Compliance:** The more extreme fasting days can be hard to adhere to, potentially leading to inconsistency.

- **Impact on Social Life:** Frequent fasting days might interfere with social activities and meal times, making it less practical for some.

Strategy for Success

- **Plan Meals Ahead:** Ensure that non-fasting days are used to consume well-balanced, nutrient-rich meals to counterbalance fasting days.

- **Monitor Energy Levels:** The way in which your body reacts to fasting days should be carefully monitored, and your activity levels should be adjusted appropriately.

4. THE EAT-STOP-EAT METHOD

The Eat-Stop-Eat approach requires participants to abstain from food for a period of twenty-four hours once or twice every week. On the other hand, if you have dinner at seven o'clock in the evening, you won't eat again until seven o'clock the following day.

Benefits for Men Over 60

- **Significant Health Benefits:** Extended fasting periods can improve metabolic health markers and enhance fat burning.

- **Increased Human Growth Hormone (HGH):** Longer fasting periods can boost HGH levels, which may help with muscle preservation and fat loss.

Drawbacks for Men Over 60

- **Intense Fasting Periods:** A 24-hour fast can be quite challenging and may lead to fatigue, dizziness, or irritability, especially for those new to fasting.

- **Potential Nutrient Deficiency:** Long fasting periods require careful planning to ensure that nutrient intake remains adequate during non-fasting periods.

Strategy for Success

- **Prepare for Fasting Days:** Ensure that the days before and after a 24-hour fast are filled with nutritious, balanced meals to support energy levels and overall health.

- **Consult a Healthcare Provider:** Given the intensity of this fasting method, it's important to get professional advice before starting.

5. THE WARRIOR DIET

The Warrior Diet entails ingesting a single, substantial meal at night, often within a four-hour eating window, and ingesting small amounts of fresh fruits and vegetables throughout the day.

Benefits for Men Over 60

- **Simplified Eating Pattern:** This method simplifies meal planning by focusing on one main meal each day.

- **Potential Weight Loss:** It is possible to lower the amount of calories consumed and to facilitate weight loss by limiting eating to a four-hour timeframe.

Drawbacks for Men Over 60

- **Hunger and Satiety Issues:** Long fasting periods during the day can lead to significant hunger, which might be difficult to manage.

- **Nutritional Adequacy:** The limited eating window requires careful planning to ensure that all nutritional needs are met within the single meal.

Strategy for Success

- **Balanced Meal Composition:** Ensure the main meal is well-balanced with adequate protein, healthy fats, and complex carbohydrates.

- **Gradual Adaptation:** Start by gradually increasing the length of the fasting period to help the body adjust.

6. TIME-RESTRICTED EATING (TRE)

Time-Restricted Eating, also known as TRE, is a method of restricting the consumption of food to a particular window of time each day. For example, you would have food between the hours of eight in the morning and four in the afternoon, and then you would abstain from eating for the other sixteen hours of the day.

Benefits for Men Over 60

- **Weight Management:** By confining eating to a set period, TRE helps reduce overall calorie consumption, which can support weight loss and management, a common concern as metabolism slows with age.

- **Improved Metabolic Health:** TRE improves insulin sensitivity and stabilizes blood sugar levels, which lowers the risk of metabolic syndrome and type 2 diabetes.

- **Simplified Routine:** TRE is straightforward to integrate into daily life, as it primarily requires adjusting meal times rather than overhauling food choices.

Drawbacks for Men Over 60

- **Initial Hunger and Adjustments:** Adapting to a new eating window can cause temporary hunger and discomfort, especially in the early stages.

- **Potential Nutritional Gaps:** If not planned properly, the restricted eating period may lead to insufficient intake of essential nutrients, which are crucial for maintaining muscle mass and bone health.

Strategy for Success

- **Gradual Implementation:** Begin with a broader eating window, such as 12 hours, and slowly reduce it to 8-10 hours as your body adapts.

- **Prioritize Balanced Meals:** Ensure that meals within the eating window are nutritionally complete, emphasizing proteins, healthy fats, and fiber-rich vegetables to support overall health and energy levels.

7. THE 12/12 METHOD

One of the most straightforward approaches to intermittent fasting is known as the 12/12 method. It entails abstaining from food for a period of twelve hours and eating only inside a window of twelve hours each day. You would eat again at seven o'clock the following morning, for example, if you finished your last meal at seven o'clock in the evening.

Benefits for Men Over 60

- **Ease of Implementation:** The 12/12 method is relatively easy to follow and doesn't require drastic changes to your daily routine.

- **Health Benefits:** Even though the fasting period is shorter, it can still improve metabolic health and support weight management.

- **Sustainable Approach:** This method is often more sustainable long-term, especially for those new to intermittent fasting or those who find longer fasting periods challenging.

Drawbacks for Men Over 60

- **Limited Impact:** The shorter fasting period may not provide as pronounced benefits as longer fasting methods in terms of metabolic health and weight loss.

- **Potential for Overeating:** The 12-hour eating window might still lead to overeating if meals are not carefully planned.

Strategy for Success

- **Balanced Meals:** Ensure that meals are nutrient-dense and well-balanced to maximize health benefits.

- **Gradual Transition:** If new to fasting, start with the 12/12 method to build tolerance before exploring more extended fasting periods.

8. THE 24-HOUR FAST

For the duration of the 24-hour fast, which is commonly performed once or twice per week, one does not consume any food for the whole day. This method is similar to Eat-Stop-Eat but focuses on a complete 24-hour period without any caloric intake.

Benefits for Men Over 60

- **Enhanced Fat Burning:** Extended fasting periods can significantly enhance fat burning and improve metabolic markers.

- **Potential Health Benefits:** Research suggests that longer fasting periods may reduce inflammation and support cardiovascular health.

Drawbacks for Men Over 60

- **Challenges with Adherence:** A full 24-hour fast can be difficult to maintain and might lead to issues such as dizziness or fatigue.

- **Nutrient Intake Concerns:** Ensuring adequate nutrient intake on non-fasting days is essential to avoid deficiencies.

Strategy for Success

- **Proper Planning:** Plan for a nutritious, balanced meal after the fasting period to replenish energy and nutrients.

- **Monitor Well-being:** Keep track of how the body responds to 24-hour fasting and adjust as necessary.

9. THE OMAD DIET (ONE MEAL A DAY)

The OMAD (One Meal a Day) diet involves consuming all daily caloric intake in a single meal each day, typically within a 1-hour eating window. The remaining 23 hours are spent fasting.

Benefits for Men Over 60

- **Simplicity:** With only one meal to plan and prepare, this approach simplifies eating patterns and can reduce meal-related stress.

- **Potential for Significant Weight Loss:** By restricting food intake to a single meal, total calorie consumption is often reduced, leading to weight loss.

Drawbacks for Men Over 60

- **Nutritional Balance:** Ensuring all essential nutrients are consumed in one meal can be challenging and may require careful planning.

- **Social and Lifestyle Impact:** The OMAD diet can impact social interactions and may be difficult to adhere to in social settings or family meals.

Strategy for Success

- **Comprehensive Meal Planning:** Focus on creating a nutritionally complete meal that includes a variety of food groups to meet daily needs.

- **Gradual Adaptation:** Start with a less restrictive eating window before transitioning to OMAD.

10. THE ALTERNATE-DAY MODIFIED FAST

The alternate-day modified fast involves fasting every other day but allows for a small amount of food (around 500-600 calories) on fasting days. This approach is less extreme than complete fasting and can be adjusted to individual needs.

Benefits for Men Over 60

- **Flexibility:** Allows for some caloric intake on fasting days, making it more manageable and less likely to cause significant fatigue or hunger.

- **Potential Health Benefits:** Provides many of the benefits of intermittent fasting while being less restrictive.

Drawbacks for Men Over 60

- **Complexity:** Managing calorie intake on fasting days while maintaining balance and nutritional adequacy can be complex.

- **Initial Adjustment:** Adapting to the alternating pattern may take time and effort.

Strategy for Success

- **Balanced Caloric Intake:** Choose nutrient-dense foods on fasting days to ensure that calorie restrictions do not lead to deficiencies.

- **Monitor Response:** It is important to pay attention to how the body reacts and to make any required adjustments to technique.

11. THE EVERY OTHER DAY DIET

The Every Other Day Diet (EOD) involves alternating days of normal eating with days of either complete fasting or very limited calorie intake (typically around 500-600 calories). This method does not prescribe specific eating windows or meal patterns, but focuses on alternating between regular eating days and fasting or very low-calorie days.

Benefits for Men Over 60

- **Weight Loss and Fat Reduction:** The significant caloric restriction on fasting days can lead to substantial weight loss and fat reduction, particularly beneficial for men struggling with weight management and abdominal fat.

- **Improved Metabolic Health:** Alternating fasting and eating days can enhance insulin sensitivity and reduce risk factors for metabolic disorders such as type 2 diabetes.

- **Flexibility:** The EOD approach offers flexibility in how one chooses to eat on regular days, which can accommodate a variety of dietary preferences and lifestyles.

Drawbacks for Men Over 60

- **Potential Nutritional Deficiencies:** On fasting or very low-calorie days, there is a risk of not meeting all nutritional needs, which can be a concern for older adults who require adequate vitamins and minerals.

- **Difficulties in Adherence:** The alternating days can make it challenging to maintain consistency and may lead to difficulties in planning and sustaining the diet long-term.

- **Initial Adjustment Issues:** Adapting to fasting every other day can cause initial issues such as fatigue, irritability, and hunger, which might be particularly pronounced in older adults.

Strategy for Success

- **Ease into the Diet:** Begin by alternating days with modified fasting, consuming around 500-600 calories on fasting days to ease your body into the routine.

- **Meal Planning:** On regular eating days, ensure meals are nutrient-dense and balanced to meet all your nutritional needs, and plan for healthy, low-calorie options on fasting days.

CONCLUSION

Individuals' health conditions and lifestyle choices can have a significant impact on whether or not they are suitable for a certain type of intermittent fasting. Each type of fasting has its own set of characteristics and potential advantages. For men over 60, it's important to choose an intermittent fasting method that aligns with their health goals, physical capabilities, and personal preferences. Whether starting with simpler approaches like the 12/12 method or exploring more complex options like OMAD, careful planning and professional guidance can help ensure a successful and healthful fasting experience.

2.4 Combining Methods for Flexibility

For men over 60, integrating or adapting intermittent fasting methods can offer a tailored approach that aligns with individual health goals, lifestyle needs, and physical capabilities. Given the diverse array of intermittent fasting strategies, combining or adjusting these methods can help address specific challenges and enhance overall effectiveness.

1. COMBINING METHODS FOR FLEXIBILITY

a. The 12/12 and 16/8 Combination: For men who are new to intermittent fasting or find the 16-hour fasting window of the 16/8 method challenging, starting with a 12-hour fast and gradually progressing to a 16-hour window can be effective. This gradual approach allows the body to adapt to longer fasting periods without significant disruption. For example, you might begin with fasting from 7 p.m. to 7 a.m. and, after a few weeks, extend the fasting period to 8 p.m. to 12 p.m. the following day. This combination offers a more manageable transition and helps ease into longer fasting windows.

b. Integrating the 5:2 Method with Time-Restricted Eating: Another effective combination involves integrating the 5:2 method with time-restricted eating techniques like the 16/8 method. On most days, follow a 16/8 fasting schedule to establish a regular eating pattern and manage weight. On the two designated fasting days, reduce calorie intake to 500-600 calories while maintaining the 16-hour fasting window. This approach balances regular eating patterns with periodic calorie restriction, potentially enhancing metabolic benefits and offering flexibility.

2. ADAPTING METHODS FOR PERSONAL NEEDS

a. Customizing the Alternate-Day Fasting (ADF): Alternate-Day Fasting can be demanding, especially for older men who may experience fatigue or difficulty adhering to complete fasting days. An adaptation involves modifying the fasting days to include a small amount of food, similar to the Alternate-Day Modified Fast. For instance, on fasting days, consume a moderate amount of calories (around 500-800) instead of a complete fast. This adaptation reduces the intensity of fasting days while still promoting the benefits of periodic calorie reduction.

b. Adjusting the Warrior Diet for Practicality: The Warrior Diet's extended fasting period can be challenging for many, particularly older adults who might struggle with long periods of minimal food intake. To adapt this method, consider shortening the eating window or incorporating a light meal or snack during the day. For example, instead of fasting from morning until evening, you could eat a small portion of high-protein, nutrient-dense foods like nuts or yogurt mid-day and have the main meal in the evening. This adjustment can help manage hunger and ensure adequate nutrient intake without compromising the diet's core principles.

2.5 Getting Started with Intermittent Fasting for Men Over 60

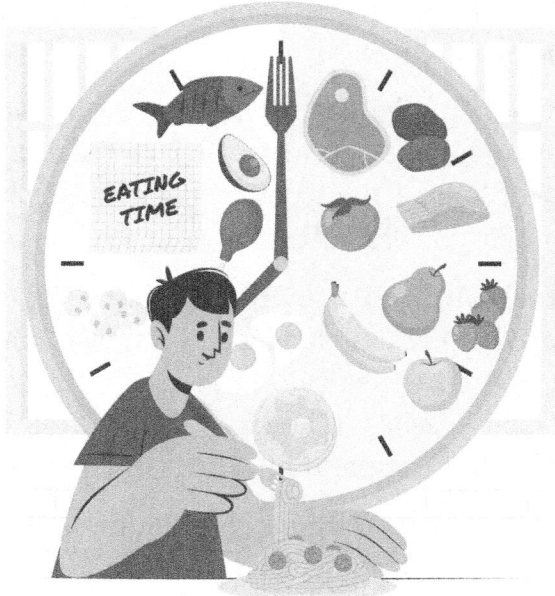

1. Set SMART Goals. Embarking on intermittent fasting can be transformative, especially for men over 60 looking to improve health and manage weight. Establishing SMART goals—Specific, Measurable, Achievable, Relevant, and Time-bound—can guide your journey and help you navigate potential challenges effectively. Consider the following aspects when setting your goals:

- **Dietary Choices**: Determine what foods and nutrients are essential during your non-fasting periods. Focus on balanced meals that support overall health and vitality.

- **Managing Symptoms**: Learn how to handle common issues like nausea or dizziness, which may arise as your body adjusts to new fasting patterns.

- **Fasting Duration**: Decide if a short-term commitment is suitable or if you're ready to embrace a longer-term fasting regimen.

- **Motivations and Current Habits**: Reflect on your reasons for fasting—whether to control blood sugar levels, lose weight, or develop healthier eating habits—and assess how current dietary habits may impact these goals. Start with simple changes, like introducing a nutritious breakfast or practicing portion control, to build a foundation for more complex fasting routines.

2. Choose a Fasting Schedule That Suits Your Lifestyle. After discussing your plans with a healthcare provider, select a fasting method that aligns with your daily routine. Consider your work schedule, sleep patterns, and personal preferences when choosing a fasting plan. Whether you opt for a shorter overnight fast or a more extended fasting period, pick a method that fits seamlessly into your lifestyle and feels practical.

3. Start Gradually. If you're new to intermittent fasting, begin with a gentle approach. Try fasting one day per week with a method that works for you. Starting with an overnight fast of 8-12 hours can help ease you into the practice. Increase the length of time you fast slowly as your body becomes accustomed to it. On days when you undertake longer fasts, choose times when you can rest and avoid strenuous activities.

4. Stay Hydrated. Hydration is crucial during fasting. Even when not consuming food, keep hydrated with non-caloric beverages such as water, herbal teas, or sparkling water. One should seek to consume a minimum of half of their body weight in oz. of water on a daily basis. For instance, if you weigh 180 pounds, you should aim to consume 90 oz. of water on a daily basis.

5. Develop a Meal Preparation Routine. Effective meal planning is essential to prevent overeating and ensure balanced nutrition during non-fasting hours. Intermittent fasting can support weight management, but excessive calorie intake during eating periods can counteract its benefits. Prepare nutrient-dense meals in advance that fit your dietary preferences—whether plant-based, low-carb, or traditional—to maintain a healthy eating pattern.

6. Focus on Balanced Nutrition. During eating windows, prioritize meals that are rich in proteins, healthy fats, and essential nutrients. This will help maintain energy levels and prolong satiety. Practice intuitive eating by paying attention to your body's signals of hunger and fullness, and steer clear of foods that are overly processed and contain an excessive amount of sugar. Eating balanced meals supports stable blood sugar levels and overall well-being.

7. Integrate Basic Nutrition Principles. Regardless of your fasting method, integrate fundamental nutrition principles such as calorie awareness and balanced eating. Whether your aim is to lose weight, enhance metabolic health, or boost energy levels, a holistic approach to nutrition will complement your intermittent fasting efforts and support your long-term health goals.

MANAGING HUNGER PANGS DURING INTERMITTENT FASTING

Hunger during fasting is triggered by ghrelin, the hormone that signals your brain when it's time to eat. Learn to differentiate between genuine hunger, which involves physical sensations like stomach growling, and cravings that may be habitual or emotional.

Strategies to Combat Hunger:

- **Stay Hydrated**: Dehydration can mimic hunger. Take in a sufficient amount of water throughout the day to prevent dehydration and to satisfy your hunger. Depending on your level of activity and the surroundings, you should aim to drink between eight and ten glasses of water every day.

- **Use Warm Liquids**: Hot beverages like tea or black coffee can help manage hunger. Opt for herbal teas or plain coffee to avoid breaking your fast. Green tea, for example, contains antioxidants that can help suppress appetite.

- **Get Enough Sleep**: Proper sleep supports hormonal balance and reduces cravings. Maintain a consistent sleep routine and create a restful environment to support your fasting goals.

- **Exercise Moderately**: Light physical activities such as walking or stretching can help distract from hunger and enhance metabolism. Gentle exercise also promotes endorphin release, which can improve mood and reduce appetite.

- **Stay Occupied**: Engaging in hobbies or activities can divert your focus from hunger. Plan activities during usual meal times to minimize feelings of deprivation. Chewing sugar-free gum can also provide a temporary distraction.

- **Implement Balanced Meals**: Focus on consuming nutrient-rich foods during eating periods. It is possible for meals that contain proteins and healthy fats to increase satiety, regulate blood sugar levels, and reduce cravings for unhealthy foods.

- **Avoid Sugary Foods and Carbs**: Limit refined sugars and carbohydrates to prevent blood sugar spikes and hunger triggers. Choose whole grains, legumes, and vegetables to maintain energy and prolong fullness.

- **Gradually Extend Fasting Hours**: Begin with shorter fasting windows and progressively extend them as your body adjusts. Align fasting hours with your natural sleep cycle to optimize benefits.

PORTION CONTROL

Effective portion control is essential for maintaining a healthy diet, especially when practicing intermittent fasting. Here are some strategies to manage portions effectively:

- **Adopt Mindful Eating**: Focus on your eating experience by eliminating distractions and savoring each bite. Mindful eating helps prevent overeating and improves digestion.

- **Use Smaller Plates**: It is possible to produce the illusion of greater portions by serving food on smaller plates, which, in turn, might help you feel content with a smaller amount of food.

- **Choose Snacks That Require Effort**: Opt for snacks that need preparation, like peeling fruit or shelling nuts. Through this procedure, you will be able to recognize indications of satiety to avoid overeating.

- **Start Meals with a Salad**: Beginning your meal with a high-fiber, low-calorie salad can curb your appetite and reduce overall calorie intake.

- **Avoid Eating Directly from Packages**: To control portions, avoid eating straight from a package. Instead, divide food into individual servings and use small containers.

- **Measure Your Portions**: Using a kitchen scale to measure portions can provide accurate servings and help manage calorie intake.

- **Drink Water Before Meals**: You may prevent yourself from overeating by drinking a glass of water before each meal. This will help you feel replete more quickly.

- **Share Meals When Dining Out**: When eating at restaurants, share large portions with others or request to have part of your meal boxed up before serving.

In conclusion, starting intermittent fasting involves careful planning and gradual adjustments. By setting clear goals, choosing a suitable fasting schedule, and implementing effective strategies for managing hunger and portion control, you can make intermittent fasting a sustainable and beneficial part of your lifestyle.

Chapter 3: Essential Foods for Men Over 60 Following IF

3.1 Recommended Foods for Intermittent Fasting

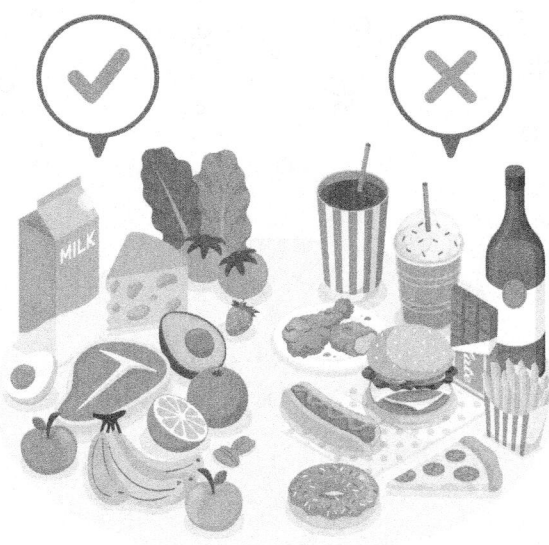

When following an intermittent fasting routine, it's crucial for men over 60 to focus on consuming nutrient-rich foods that support overall health and well-being. Prioritizing lean proteins is especially important, as they help maintain satiety for longer periods and contribute to muscle preservation, which is vital as we age. Opt for lean protein sources such as plain Greek yogurt, skinless chicken breast, fish, seafood, beans, lentils, tofu, and tempeh. These proteins not only promote fullness but also help support muscle maintenance, which becomes increasingly important in later years. Including a variety of fruits and vegetables in your diet is also key to a successful intermittent fasting plan. These natural foods are packed with essential vitamins, minerals, and fiber, all of which play a crucial role in promoting digestive health, regulating blood sugar levels, and managing cholesterol. Moreover, most fruits and vegetables are low in calories, making them excellent choices for your eating windows during intermittent fasting. Recommended fruits for men over 60 include apples, apricots, berries (such as blackberries and blueberries), cherries, pears, plums, melons, and oranges. These fruits are nutrient-dense and can provide natural sweetness while supporting your overall health. Vegetables are another cornerstone of a balanced intermittent fasting diet. Leafy greens, in particular, offer substantial health benefits, including supporting heart health, reducing the risk of chronic diseases like type 2 diabetes, and promoting cognitive function. Eating a diet rich in vegetables can help protect against age-related diseases, making them an essential part of your daily intake. According to dietary guidelines, men should aim for almost 2.5 cups of vegetables daily, especially when following a 2,000-calorie diet. Affordable, nutrient-packed vegetables such as broccoli, carrots, cauliflower, tomatoes, and green beans should be staples in your meal planning. Leafy greens like spinach, kale, arugula, cabbage, and chard are particularly beneficial due to their high fiber content and the abundance of vitamins they offer.

3.2 Suggested Food Items for Intermittent Fasting

This list provides a starting point for foods that align well with intermittent fasting, particularly for men over 60. It's important to remember that this is not a comprehensive list. You can adapt and expand it based on your individual tastes and nutritional needs. Prioritize whole, nutrient-dense foods that will support both your overall health and your intermittent fasting objectives.

Lean Proteins:

- ✓ Chicken breast
- ✓ Turkey
- ✓ Fish (salmon, tuna, cod, etc.)
- ✓ Shellfish (shrimp, crab, mussels, etc.)
- ✓ Lean cuts of beef or pork
- ✓ Eggs
- ✓ Tofu and tempeh

Fruits:

- ✓ Apples
- ✓ Berries (blueberries, strawberries, raspberries, etc.)
- ✓ Citrus fruits (oranges, grapefruits, lemons, etc.)
- ✓ Apricots
- ✓ Pears
- ✓ Peaches
- ✓ Plums
- ✓ Melons (watermelon, cantaloupe, honeydew)

Vegetables:

- ✓ Broccoli
- ✓ Cauliflower
- ✓ Spinach
- ✓ Kale
- ✓ Tomatoes
- ✓ Carrots
- ✓ Bell peppers
- ✓ Cucumbers
- ✓ Zucchini
- ✓ Green beans

Healthy Fats:

- • Avocado
- • Nuts (almonds, walnuts, pistachios, etc.)
- • Seeds (chia seeds, flaxseeds, pumpkin seeds, etc.)
- • Olive oil
- • Coconut oil
- • Avocado oil

Beverages:

- • Water (plain or infused with fruits/herbs)
- • Herbal teas (peppermint, chamomile, ginger, etc.)
- • Black coffee (without added sugar or cream)
- • Green tea

Condiments and Spices:

- Fresh herbs (parsley, basil, cilantro, etc.)
- Garlic and ginger
- Turmeric
- Cinnamon
- Chili flakes
- Mustard
- Apple cider vinegar

Healthy Carbohydrates:

- Sweet potatoes
- Quinoa
- Brown rice
- Oats (steel-cut or rolled)
- Whole-grain bread (in moderation)
- Lentils
- Chickpeas

Dairy (if tolerated):

- Greek yogurt (plain, unsweetened)
- Cottage cheese

Non-Dairy Alternatives:

- Almond milk (unsweetened)
- Coconut milk (unsweetened)

Healthy Snacks:

- Raw nuts and seeds (portion-controlled)
- Nut butter (almond, peanut, etc.)
- Hummus with raw vegetables
- Rice cakes (whole-grain)
- Popcorn (air-popped, without added butter or excessive salt)

Low-Calorie Foods:

- Cabbage
- Cauliflower rice
- Zucchini noodles (zoodles)
- Mushrooms
- Brussels sprouts

Probiotic Foods:

- Kimchi
- Sauerkraut
- Yogurt with live cultures (if tolerated)

Remember to be mindful of portion sizes and balance your meals with a variety of nutrient-dense foods. It's essential to listen to your body's hunger and fullness cues and make adjustments as needed. Please consult with a healthcare professional or a registered dietitian if you have specific dietary concerns or medical conditions.

3.3 Foods to Limit on an Intermittent Fasting Diet

When adhering to an intermittent fasting regimen, it's important to be mindful of certain foods that can undermine your efforts. Foods high in calories, saturated fats, and sodium not only offer little nutritional value but can also cause spikes in hunger, defeating the purpose of fasting. These foods often lack the necessary nutrients to sustain your energy and health, especially for men over 60 who may need to focus on heart health, maintaining muscle mass, and managing weight.

To maintain a successful intermittent fasting schedule, limit or avoid the following:

- **Processed Snack Foods:** Items like chips and other packaged snacks are typically high in unhealthy fats and calories, offering little nutritional benefit.

- **Refined Grains:** Pretzels, crackers, and other refined grain products often lack essential nutrients and may contain additives that could disrupt your health goals.

- **Sugary Foods and Drinks:** Foods with added sugars, such as candy, pastries, sugary cereals, and sweetened beverages, offer empty calories that can lead to energy crashes and cravings. Limiting these will help maintain steady energy levels and reduce unnecessary calorie intake.

By focusing on whole, nutrient-dense foods and being aware of what to avoid, you can make intermittent fasting a more effective and sustainable approach to improving your overall health. Always consult with a healthcare provider to ensure that your dietary choices align with your individual health needs and conditions.

3.4 Integrating Traditional Medicine and Natural Remedies with Intermittent Fasting for Men Over 60

Combining traditional medicine and natural remedies with intermittent fasting can offer a more comprehensive approach to maintaining health, especially for men over 60. This integration can help enhance the benefits of fasting, support the management of chronic conditions, and promote overall wellness. Here's how to incorporate these approaches effectively.

Understanding Traditional Medicine

Traditional medicine includes practices such as herbal remedies, acupuncture, Ayurveda, and Traditional Chinese Medicine (TCM). These methods focus on restoring balance in the body, which complements the benefits of intermittent fasting.

- **Herbal Medicine:** Using plant-based remedies can support digestion, metabolism, and organ function, which are essential during fasting periods. For instance, ginger is well-known for its anti-inflammatory and digestive benefits, helping to alleviate any discomfort associated with fasting. Turmeric, with its powerful anti-inflammatory and antioxidant properties, supports overall health and can reduce inflammation. Green tea, rich in antioxidants, boosts metabolism and aids weight management, making it an excellent addition to fasting periods.

However, it's crucial to consult with your healthcare provider to ensure that any herbal remedies you use don't interact negatively with your current medications or health conditions.

- **Acupuncture:** A key component of TCM, acupuncture involves the strategic placement of thin needles at specific points on the body to balance energy flow, or Qi. For men over 60, acupuncture can help alleviate side effects of fasting such as headaches, fatigue, and digestive issues. Additionally, acupuncture can promote overall well-being by reducing stress, improving sleep, and increasing energy levels.

- **Ayurveda:** This ancient Indian system of medicine emphasizes balance within the body's systems through diet, herbal remedies, and breathing exercises. By aligning your dietary choices with your Ayurvedic body type (Vata, Pitta, Kapha), you can optimize the health benefits of intermittent fasting.

Natural Remedies

Natural remedies often overlap with traditional medicine and include dietary supplements, essential oils, and homeopathic treatments. These remedies can support health during fasting by addressing specific needs.

- **Dietary Supplements:** Intermittent fasting can enhance nutrient absorption, but it's still important to ensure adequate intake of key vitamins and minerals, especially for men over 60. Consider multivitamins to cover nutritional gaps, omega-3 fatty acids for heart health and cognitive function, and vitamin D and calcium for bone strength. Always consult your healthcare provider before starting any new supplements to avoid potential interactions with your current medications.

- **Essential Oils:** Essential oils offer various health benefits, such as reducing stress, improving digestion, and enhancing sleep. For example, lavender can help with relaxation and sleep, peppermint can support digestion and alleviate headaches, and lemon can boost energy and improve mood. These oils can be used in diffusers, added to baths, or applied topically with a carrier oil.

Integrating Practices for a Holistic Approach

To successfully integrate traditional medicine and natural remedies with intermittent fasting, it's important to start with a discussion with your healthcare provider. Review any new treatments with a professional to ensure they complement your current health status and medications. Every individual's health needs and tolerances are unique, so tailor the integration of these practices to your specific situation. Monitor your health regularly and adjust your approach as necessary, paying attention to changes in symptoms, energy levels, and overall well-being.

A balanced approach is key—avoid over-reliance on any single method. Strive for a holistic routine that includes a healthy diet, regular physical activity, mental wellness, and a combination of traditional or natural remedies. Stay informed about the benefits and risks of different traditional medicines and natural treatments, relying on credible sources and professional advice to make educated decisions.

Integrating traditional medicine and natural remedies with intermittent fasting can significantly enhance the benefits of fasting and support overall health, particularly for men over 60. By carefully planning and consulting healthcare providers, you can adopt a more holistic approach to health that balances the wisdom of ancient practices with modern insights.

3.5 Evaluating the Safety and Effectiveness of Supplements for Men Over 60

As men over 60 explore the benefits of intermittent fasting, it's important to carefully evaluate the supplements they might incorporate into their lifestyle. As we age, our bodies become more susceptible to nutrient deficiencies and imbalances, making it essential to approach supplementation thoughtfully. When selecting supplements, quality is key. Choosing products that have been tested for purity and effectiveness is crucial. Certifications from third-party organizations like NSF International, ConsumerLab, or the US Pharmacopeia (USP) are reliable indicators that the supplement meets strict standards and contains what it claims to, without harmful contaminants. In addition to choosing high-quality products, it's important to understand the active ingredients in supplements. Knowing what these ingredients do and how they interact with other nutrients and medications helps determine whether they are appropriate for your needs. For instance, calcium is essential for bone health, but taking too much can cause problems like kidney stones or interfere with other minerals like magnesium. Similarly, while vitamin D supports calcium absorption, excessive amounts can lead to toxicity.

Scientific research can also provide valuable insight into a supplement's effectiveness. It's wise to rely on peer-reviewed studies and trusted sources like academic journals and government health websites, rather than anecdotal evidence or testimonials, which may not give a complete picture of a supplement's benefits. Additionally, understanding potential side effects and interactions with medications is critical. Some supplements can have adverse effects or interfere with prescription medications. For example, St. John's Wort, a popular supplement for managing depression, can reduce the effectiveness of blood thinners and other medications. Reading labels and discussing potential risks with your healthcare provider can help prevent unwanted complications.

Dosage is another essential factor in supplement safety. More is not always better, and taking supplements in excessive amounts can lead to toxicity or other health problems. It's important to follow the recommended dosage on the label or as advised by a healthcare professional, starting with the lowest effective dose and adjusting as needed. Monitoring your body's response to supplements is also crucial. Regularly assess any changes in your health, both positive and negative, and share this information with your healthcare provider. Routine check-ups can help determine if the supplements are working as expected or if any adjustments need to be made.

While supplements can be beneficial, they should not replace a balanced diet. Whole foods offer a complex array of nutrients that work together in ways that supplements alone cannot replicate. Emphasizing a diet rich in fruits, vegetables, lean proteins, whole grains, and healthy fats will provide most of the nutrients needed to support overall health. Supplements should present as a complement to a nutritious diet, filling in any gaps where needed.

Chapter 4: Digital Health Tools and Trusted Resources for Men Over 60

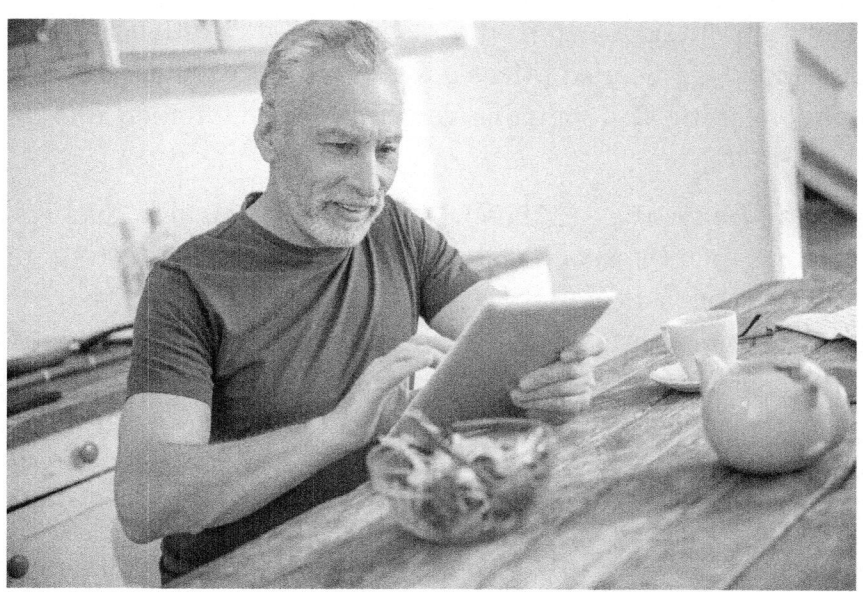

4.1 Reliable Websites

For men over 60, health management requires a combination of accurate information and practical tools to support daily decision-making. Reliable websites and communities can present as vital resources in navigating the complexities of aging, intermittent fasting, and maintaining overall wellness. However, it's essential to approach online information with a critical eye, ensuring that the sources consulted are credible, evidence-based, and relevant to individual health needs. Websites affiliated with reputable medical institutions, government health agencies, and nonprofit organizations dedicated to senior health tend to offer the most reliable information. There are several websites dedicated to the health of older adults, offering medically reviewed information on a wide range of topics. These platforms are particularly valuable for men over 60 as they address common health challenges associated with aging, such as heart disease, diabetes, prostate health, and maintaining physical strength and vitality. The following are examples of trustworthy websites that provide comprehensive and evidence-based health advice:

- **National Institute on Aging (NIA).** The National Institute on Aging, part of the U.S. National Institutes of Health, offers a wealth of information on healthy aging. Their website provides research-backed articles on topics relevant to men over 60, including managing chronic conditions, nutrition, and physical activity. NIA also offers guidance on mental health and cognitive function, which are critical components of aging well. This site is a reliable source for understanding how intermittent fasting may interact with age-related conditions, and it frequently updates its resources based on the latest scientific findings.

- **Mayo Clinic.** The Mayo Clinic is one of the most respected medical institutions globally, and its website offers detailed, easy-to-understand health information. For men over 60, the Mayo Clinic provides articles on managing heart health, controlling blood sugar, and maintaining mobility—all of which are critical when adopting an intermittent fasting lifestyle. Their content is written and reviewed by healthcare professionals, ensuring accuracy. The Mayo Clinic also offers a symptom checker and a variety of tools to help monitor health, making it a valuable resource for older men looking to stay proactive about their well-being.

- **Men's Health Network (MHN).** The Men's Health Network is a nonprofit organization that focuses specifically on health issues affecting men. Their website provides resources on a broad spectrum of topics, from preventive care to managing chronic diseases. For men over 60 practicing intermittent fasting, MHN offers insights into how to balance fasting with the need for nutrient-dense foods, especially in managing conditions like hypertension and diabetes. This platform also emphasizes the importance of mental health, offering resources on dealing with stress, depression, and anxiety in later life.

- **American Heart Association (AHA).** Cardiovascular health is a major concern for men over 60, and the American Heart Association offers authoritative advice on maintaining heart health. Their website includes information on heart-friendly diets, physical activity guidelines, and how intermittent fasting might affect cardiovascular risk factors like blood pressure and cholesterol. The AHA also provides helpful tools, such as meal planning guides and fitness trackers, to support heart health in a practical, actionable way.

- **AARP (American Association of Retired Persons).** AARP is a well-known organization that advocates for people over 50, and their website offers a robust health section with articles tailored to the needs of older adults. For men over 60, AARP provides resources on maintaining a healthy weight, managing chronic conditions, and understanding how lifestyle choices, such as intermittent fasting, can impact overall health. They also have a vibrant community section where older adults can connect and share experiences, which can be incredibly supportive for those exploring fasting and other wellness practices.

4.2 Online Communities and Support Forums

Navigating health challenges and lifestyle changes, such as intermittent fasting, can be more manageable with the support of a community. Several online forums and communities provide a space for men over 60 to connect, share experiences, and seek advice. These platforms are especially beneficial for those who may not have access to local support groups or prefer the convenience of online interaction.

- **Reddit – r/IntermittentFasting.** Reddit's Intermittent Fasting subreddit has a large and active community where users share their experiences, challenges, and successes with fasting. For men over 60, this forum offers a wealth of first-hand advice, including how to adjust fasting schedules to suit specific health conditions and how to maintain muscle mass and energy levels. While the forum is open to all ages, there are often discussions tailored to older adults, making it a supportive environment for seniors exploring fasting.

- **Men's Health Network Community.** The Men's Health Network not only provides informative articles but also hosts community forums where men can discuss various health issues, including intermittent fasting. These forums are moderated, ensuring that discussions stay on topic and that the information shared is respectful and supportive. Men over 60 can benefit from the camaraderie and shared knowledge of others facing similar health challenges and lifestyle changes.

- **AARP Online Community.** The AARP online community offers discussion boards on a wide range of topics, including health and wellness. Men over 60 can find specific threads related to intermittent fasting, aging, and managing chronic conditions. The AARP community is particularly beneficial for those seeking advice from peers who understand the unique health challenges that come with aging.

4.3 Recommended Academic Journals for Men Over 60

For men over 60 who are dedicated to maintaining their health and well-being, staying informed through credible, research-based sources is essential. Academic journals provide access to the latest studies and reviews on health, aging, nutrition, and intermittent fasting. Unlike popular media, academic journals undergo rigorous peer-review processes, ensuring that the information is scientifically valid and trustworthy. For older men practicing intermittent fasting, these journals can offer valuable insights into how diet, fasting, and lifestyle choices affect health as they age. Below are several highly respected academic journals that focus on topics relevant to men over 60.

- **THE JOURNAL OF GERONTOLOGY SERIES A: BIOLOGICAL SCIENCES AND MEDICAL SCIENCES.** This journal is one of the most respected publications in the field of aging. It covers a broad range of topics related to the biology of aging, clinical medicine, and age-related health conditions. For men over 60, this journal is particularly valuable as it provides cutting-edge research on the physical and biological changes that occur with age. Articles often address how diet and lifestyle choices, including intermittent fasting, can impact longevity, cognitive health, and chronic disease management. Studies published here can provide insights into how fasting might influence cellular aging, muscle preservation, and cardiovascular health in older men.

■ **AGE AND AGEING.** Published by Oxford University Press, AGE AND AGEING is a leading journal in geriatric medicine. This journal focuses on clinical aspects of aging and provides practical advice on managing age-related conditions. It includes research on nutrition, physical activity, and overall health strategies for older adults. For men over 60, this journal is an excellent resource for understanding how intermittent fasting may interact with conditions like diabetes, hypertension, and arthritis. The journal often features articles on the best practices for healthy aging, providing actionable insights into maintaining vitality and well-being in later years.

■ **NUTRITION AND HEALTHY AGING.** This journal specifically addresses the intersection of diet, nutrition, and aging. For men over 60, NUTRITION AND HEALTHY AGING offers valuable research on how dietary patterns, including intermittent fasting, can affect health outcomes. Topics such as muscle mass preservation, nutrient absorption, and metabolic health are frequently discussed, making it a key resource for those interested in how nutrition influences aging. The journal also explores how intermittent fasting can be adapted to meet the nutritional needs of older adults, ensuring that fasting supports rather than detracts from overall health.

■ **THE AMERICAN JOURNAL OF CLINICAL NUTRITION.** As one of the leading journals in the field of nutrition, THE AMERICAN JOURNAL OF CLINICAL NUTRITION provides a wealth of information on how dietary choices impact health across the lifespan. For older men practicing intermittent fasting, this journal offers research on how different eating patterns affect metabolic health, weight management, and the prevention of chronic diseases. Studies in this journal often examine the long-term effects of various diets, including fasting, on heart health, diabetes, and cognitive function—key concerns for men over 60.

■ **THE JOURNALS OF GERONTOLOGY: PSYCHOLOGICAL SCIENCES AND SOCIAL SCIENCES.** This journal focuses on the psychological and social aspects of aging, which are crucial for maintaining mental health and a positive outlook in later life. For men over 60, understanding the psychological effects of intermittent fasting, such as changes in mood, energy levels, and cognitive function, is essential. The journal also explores the social dynamics of aging, including how relationships and community engagement can impact health. Articles from this journal can provide insights into how fasting influences not just physical health, but also mental and emotional well-being.

■ **THE JOURNAL OF AGING AND PHYSICAL ACTIVITY.** Physical activity is a key component of healthy aging, and this journal specializes in research on exercise and physical activity in older adults. For men over 60, combining intermittent fasting with an active lifestyle can be a powerful way to enhance health. THE JOURNAL OF AGING AND PHYSICAL ACTIVITY publishes studies on how exercise can help mitigate the effects of aging, maintain muscle mass, and improve cardiovascular health—all of which are important for those practicing intermittent fasting. This journal also examines how fasting affects exercise performance and recovery in older adults, providing practical guidance for integrating fasting with fitness.

- DIABETES CARE. For men over 60, managing blood sugar levels is often a critical concern, especially if they are practicing intermittent fasting. DIABETES CARE is a leading journal that focuses on the latest research in diabetes management, prevention, and treatment. For those dealing with prediabetes or type 2 diabetes, understanding how intermittent fasting can influence blood glucose levels and insulin sensitivity is crucial. This journal provides in-depth studies on how different fasting protocols impact diabetes management, offering evidence-based guidance for older men looking to control their blood sugar through dietary interventions.

- JOURNAL OF THE AMERICAN GERIATRICS SOCIETY. The JOURNAL OF THE AMERICAN GERIATRICS SOCIETY (JAGS) is a top resource for clinical care and research related to older adults. This journal publishes studies on a wide range of topics, including nutrition, cognitive health, and chronic disease management. For men over 60, JAGS provides critical insights into how intermittent fasting can be safely integrated into a comprehensive health plan, particularly when managing multiple health conditions. The journal frequently covers the latest in geriatric medicine, offering practical advice on how to balance fasting with other health priorities, such as medication management and dietary supplementation.

4.4 Digital Tools and Apps for Health and Wellness Monitoring

Incorporating digital tools and apps into daily routines can be a game changer for men over 60 who are practicing intermittent fasting. These tools not only simplify the process of tracking fasting windows, meals, and physical activity, but they also provide insights into key health metrics like blood sugar, blood pressure, and overall nutrition. In addition to tracking physical health, digital tools that promote mindfulness and stress management can significantly contribute to overall well-being.

Fasting and Nutrition Tracking Apps

- **Zero** is a highly recommended app for intermittent fasting. It allows users to customize their fasting windows, track progress, and access educational content tailored to different fasting methods. For men over 60, Zero's ability to integrate with other health apps and wearables can help monitor how fasting impacts health over time.

- **MyFitnessPal** is a comprehensive nutrition tracking app that helps users log food intake, monitor caloric consumption, and understand nutrient breakdowns. This is particularly useful for older adults to ensure that they are getting adequate nutrition during non-fasting periods.

- **Lifesum** combines food tracking with intermittent fasting schedules, helping users plan meals that align with their fasting goals. The app also offers personalized meal plans, making it easier to focus on nutrient-dense foods that support healthy aging.

Health Monitoring Apps

- **Blood Pressure Companion** is an easy-to-use app for tracking blood pressure readings, making it ideal for older men managing hypertension. Keeping a detailed record of blood pressure changes while practicing intermittent fasting can help identify patterns and adjust diet and lifestyle accordingly.

- **Glucose Buddy** is designed for individuals managing diabetes or prediabetes. It tracks blood glucose levels, insulin usage, and meals. This app is especially valuable for men over 60 who need to monitor how intermittent fasting affects their blood sugar levels and overall glucose management.

- **Apple Health** and **Google Fit** offer a wide range of health monitoring capabilities. These apps can track steps, sleep, activity levels, and even integrate with other health devices like blood pressure monitors and glucose trackers. For men over 60, these tools provide a centralized way to monitor overall health metrics and see how fasting fits into the bigger picture of wellness.

Mindfulness and Stress Management Apps

- **Headspace** is a popular mindfulness app that offers guided meditations and breathing exercises to help manage stress and improve mental clarity. For older adults, maintaining mental well-being is just as important as physical health, especially when adopting a new lifestyle like intermittent fasting.

- **Calm** provides a variety of meditation programs focused on stress reduction, sleep improvement, and mindfulness. Regular use of such apps can help reduce fasting-related stress and promote relaxation.

- **Insight Timer** offers thousands of free guided meditations and mindfulness practices. Men over 60 can benefit from using these tools to manage stress, improve focus, and foster a sense of calm during fasting periods.

4.5 Resources for Managing Chronic Conditions

Managing chronic health conditions is a significant concern for men over 60, and intermittent fasting can offer benefits when carefully integrated with other health strategies. Digital resources and platforms can provide the necessary support for managing conditions like type 2 diabetes, hypertension, and cardiovascular diseases. Below are some key resources to help older men navigate their health while incorporating intermittent fasting into their daily routines.

Diabetes Management

- **MySugr** is an app designed to make diabetes management easier and more engaging. It allows users to track blood sugar levels, insulin intake, and food consumption. MySugr also offers personalized insights and reports that can help older men see how intermittent fasting is affecting their glucose control over time.

- **BlueLoop** by the College Diabetes Network is another useful platform that supports individuals with diabetes. It offers a secure space for logging and sharing diabetes-related data with healthcare providers, making it easier to manage the condition while following a fasting regimen.

Hypertension and Cardiovascular Health

- **HeartWise Blood Pressure Tracker** is an app specifically designed to help individuals monitor their blood pressure and heart rate. Older men who are practicing intermittent fasting can use this app to track changes in cardiovascular health and ensure their fasting routine supports heart health.

- **CardioSmart** is a patient education website by the American College of Cardiology that offers resources for managing cardiovascular conditions. It provides practical advice, tools, and resources tailored to heart health, including guidance on diet and exercise, which can be aligned with intermittent fasting practices.

General Chronic Disease Management

- **CareZone** is a comprehensive app that helps manage medications, doctor's appointments, and health records. This app is particularly useful for older adults with multiple chronic conditions. By keeping all health-related information in one place, CareZone simplifies the process of managing fasting alongside other treatments.

- **Medisafe** is another medication management app that helps users stay on top of their prescriptions and supplements. For men over 60 practicing intermittent fasting, staying consistent with medications is critical, and Medisafe can ensure that fasting windows don't interfere with essential treatments.

Online Platforms and Support Communities

- **HealthUnlocked** is an online community where individuals with chronic conditions can connect, share experiences, and access information. There are forums dedicated to specific conditions like diabetes, hypertension, and heart disease, where older men can learn from others who are managing similar challenges while following intermittent fasting.

- **PatientsLikeMe** is a platform that allows users to track their health, connect with others who share similar conditions, and gain insights from real-world experiences. For men over 60 with chronic conditions, this resource can offer support and advice on balancing intermittent fasting with their health needs.

By leveraging these digital tools and resources, men over 60 can better manage their health while practicing intermittent fasting. These apps and platforms not only help track vital health metrics but also offer support and education to ensure that fasting is done safely and effectively, enhancing both physical and mental well-being.

Chapter 5: Exercise and Intermittent Fasting for Men Over 60

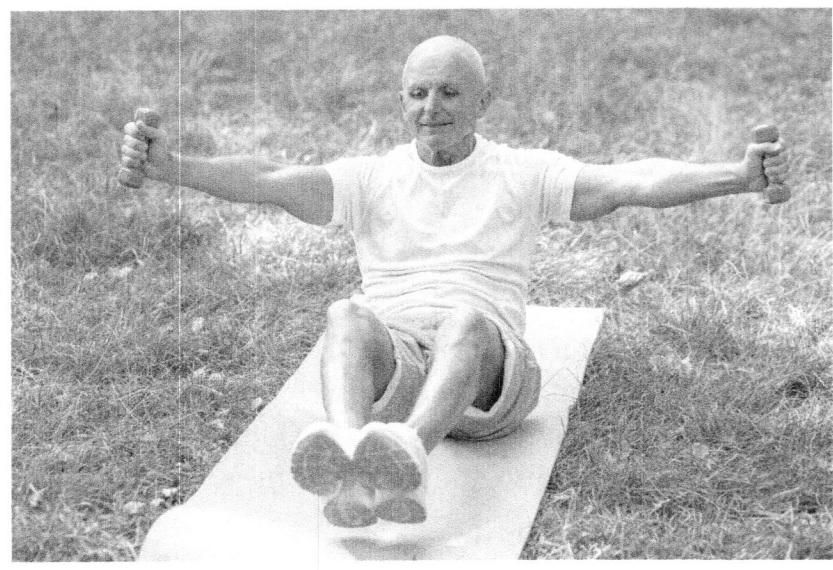

5.1 The Synergy of IFand Physical Activity for Men Over 60

Integrating intermittent fasting with regular physical activity can be especially beneficial for men over 60, offering a comprehensive approach to enhancing overall health and well-being. As men age, maintaining a healthy lifestyle becomes increasingly important to manage weight, support cardiovascular health, and preserve muscle mass. Combining these two strategies—intermittent fasting and exercise—can create a powerful synergy that promotes healthy aging and improves quality of life. For men over 60, exercise offers numerous benefits, including enhanced cardiovascular health, improved bone density, and better mental well-being. Engaging in both aerobic and resistance exercises can help address common age-related issues such as muscle loss, decreased bone density, and reduced cardiovascular fitness.

Aerobic exercise, such as walking, swimming, or cycling, is essential for maintaining heart health. It improves cardiovascular fitness, lowers blood pressure, and helps regulate cholesterol levels. For older men, aiming for almost 150 minutes of moderate-intensity aerobic exercise per week can significantly reduce the risk of heart disease and stroke.

Resistance training, which includes activities like weight lifting or bodyweight exercises, is crucial for preserving and building muscle mass. As men age, muscle mass naturally decreases, a condition known as sarcopenia. Resistance training helps combat this loss, improving strength, balance, and functional capacity. It also supports bone health by enhancing bone density, which is important for preventing osteoporosis and fractures.

The combination of intermittent fasting and physical activity can amplify the benefits of both approaches. Here's how integrating these strategies can enhance overall health:

Optimized Fat Loss and Muscle Preservation: Exercising during fasting periods can enhance fat burning and improve metabolic health. When the body is in a fasted state, it is more likely to use stored fat as an energy source. Combining this with resistance training ensures that while fat is being burned, muscle mass is maintained or even increased.

- **Improved Insulin Sensitivity**: Both intermittent fasting and regular exercise have positive effects on insulin sensitivity. When used together, they can significantly improve the body's ability to manage blood sugar levels. This is especially important for men over 60, who may be at higher risk for developing insulin resistance.

- **Enhanced Cellular Repair and Recovery**: Exercise increases oxidative stress, which can lead to cellular damage. Intermittent fasting supports autophagy, the body's natural process of repairing and regenerating cells. The combination of fasting and exercise can therefore enhance recovery and promote healthier aging by facilitating more effective cellular repair.

- **Balanced Energy Levels**: Intermittent fasting can help regulate energy levels throughout the day. When combined with physical activity, it ensures that energy levels are optimal for workouts and daily activities. Exercising during the eating window can provide the necessary fuel for performance, while fasting periods allow the body to rest and repair.

Practical Tips for Combining Intermittent Fasting and Exercise

- **Timing Your Workouts**: For many men over 60, working out during the eating window can be more effective, as the body has access to energy from recent meals. However, some may prefer exercising in a fasted state. It's important to listen to your body and find a routine that works best for you.

- **Hydration and Nutrition**: Staying hydrated is crucial, especially when combining fasting with exercise. Drink plenty of water throughout the day, and ensure you're consuming adequate electrolytes. During eating periods, focus on nutrient-dense foods that provide the necessary vitamins, minerals, and protein to support your exercise routine.

- **Gradual Integration**: If you're new to either intermittent fasting or exercise, start gradually. Begin with shorter fasting periods and lighter exercise routines, and progressively increase intensity and duration as your body adapts.

- **Consult with Professionals**: Before starting any new exercise or fasting regimen, consult with a healthcare provider or a fitness professional. They can help tailor a plan to your specific health needs and ensure that both fasting and exercise are appropriate for your individual health status.

5.2 Precautions for Physical Activity in Men Over 60 Practicing Intermittent Fasting

When men over 60 incorporate intermittent fasting (IF) into their lifestyle, it's essential to approach physical activity with particular care. Combining IF with exercise can offer substantial health benefits, but it also requires careful planning to ensure safety and effectiveness. Here are key precautions to consider to optimize the benefits of both intermittent fasting and physical activity while minimizing risks.

1. Understanding Your Body's Signals

As we age, the body's response to physical activity can change, and this is further influenced by intermittent fasting. Men over 60 should pay close attention to their body's signals during exercise.

Signs of excessive fatigue, dizziness, or discomfort may indicate that the body is struggling to cope with the combined demands of fasting and exercise. Listening to these signals and adjusting your routine accordingly can help prevent overtraining and injury. The timing of physical activity in relation to fasting periods can significantly impact performance and safety. Many men find that exercising during the eating window allows them to perform at their best, as the body has adequate fuel for energy. Conversely, working out during fasting periods might lead to decreased performance and increased risk of dehydration or muscle breakdown.

When engaging in physical activity, consider the following:

- **Low to Moderate Intensity**: If exercising during a fasted state, opt for lower intensity activities such as walking or gentle stretching. High-intensity workouts might be better suited to when you have recently eaten, as they require more immediate energy.

- **Adjust Intensity Gradually**: Start with moderate exercises and gradually increase the intensity based on your body's response and tolerance. Avoid sudden or extreme changes in workout routines that can lead to injury.

2. Hydration and Electrolyte Balance

Proper hydration is crucial, especially when combining fasting with exercise. Dehydration can impair physical performance and recovery, and fasting may increase the risk of dehydration if fluid intake is insufficient. To maintain optimal hydration:

- **Drink Water Regularly**: Ensure you are drinking water throughout the day, not just during or after exercise. During fasting periods, consume fluids like water and herbal teas to stay hydrated.

- **Consider Electrolytes**: If engaging in prolonged or intense workouts, consider incorporating electrolyte-rich drinks to replenish lost sodium, potassium, and magnesium.

3. Nutritional Support

During fasting periods, it's important to ensure that nutrient intake meets your physical needs. Nutritional support plays a key role in optimizing energy levels and recovery.

- **Balanced Meals**: During eating windows, focus on balanced meals that provide a mix of protein, carbohydrates, healthy fats, and micronutrients to support exercise and recovery. Adequate protein intake is especially important for muscle repair and growth.

- **Pre-Workout Nutrition**: If you plan to exercise shortly after eating, include a combination of carbohydrates and protein to fuel your workout and enhance performance.

4. Adjusting to Individual Health Conditions

Men over 60 often have specific health conditions that may affect their ability to exercise safely. It's crucial to take these conditions into account when planning physical activities.

- **Consult Healthcare Providers**: Before beginning any new exercise routine or fasting regimen, consult with a healthcare provider to ensure that both are appropriate for your health status and any existing conditions.

- **Personalize Exercise Routines**: Work with a fitness professional to create a customized exercise plan that accommodates any health issues or physical limitations. For instance, men with joint problems might benefit from low-impact activities like swimming or cycling.

5. Gradual Integration and Monitoring

Integrating intermittent fasting with a new exercise routine should be done gradually. Sudden or drastic changes can lead to adverse effects, such as excessive fatigue or injury.

- **Start Slowly**: Begin with shorter, less intense workouts and gradually increase both duration and intensity. Monitor how your body responds to these changes and adjust as necessary.

- **Regular Monitoring**: Keep track of your energy levels, recovery times, and overall well-being. If you notice any negative effects or significant changes in health, consult with a healthcare provider.

6. Recovery and Rest

Proper recovery is essential when combining intermittent fasting with physical activity. Adequate rest and recovery help prevent overtraining and support muscle repair and overall health.

- **Prioritize Rest**: Ensure you get enough sleep and allow for rest days between intense workout sessions. Quality sleep supports recovery and overall health.

- **Active Recovery**: Incorporate gentle activities like walking or stretching on rest days to promote circulation and reduce muscle stiffness.

5.3 28-Day Exercise Plan for Men Over 60 (Compatible with IF Lifestyle)

This 28-day exercise plan is designed to provide a balanced approach to fitness for men over 60 who are practicing intermittent fasting. It incorporates a mix of cardiovascular, strength, flexibility, and balance exercises to support overall health while aligning with the fasting lifestyle. The plan includes rest days to ensure adequate recovery. Adjustments can be made based on individual fitness levels and health conditions.

DAY 1: CARDIOVASCULAR EXERCISE

Activity: Brisk Walking
Duration: 30 minutes
How to Perform: Walk at a pace where you can talk but not sing. Ensure your posture is upright, with a slight lean forward and your arms swinging naturally.

DAY 2: STRENGTH TRAINING (UPPER BODY)

Activity: Seated Dumbbell Press
Duration: 3 sets of 12 reps
How to Perform: Sit on a chair with back support, hold a dumbbell in each hand at shoulder height, and press upwards until arms are fully extended. Lower the weights back to shoulder height.

DAY 3: FLEXIBILITY AND BALANCE

Activity: Gentle Yoga

Duration: 30 minutes

How to Perform: Focus on gentle stretches and balance poses such as the Tree Pose and Warrior I. Use a chair or wall for support if

DAY 4: REST DAY

needed.

DAY 5: CARDIOVASCULAR EXERCISE

Cycling
Duration: 30 minutes
How to Perform: Ride a stationary bike or a regular bike at a moderate pace. Adjust the seat height to ensure proper leg extension.

DAY 7: REST DAY

DAY 6: STRENGTH TRAINING (LOWER BODY)

Chair Squats
Duration: 3 sets of 12 reps
How to Perform: Stand in front of a chair with feet hip-width apart. Lower yourself as if sitting down, touch the chair lightly, and then stand back up.

DAY 8: CARDIOVASCULAR EXERCISE

Swimming or Water Aerobics
Duration: 30 minutes
How to Perform: Swim laps at a moderate pace or participate in a water aerobics class. Use the water's resistance to enhance the workout while minimizing joint stress.

DAY 9: STRENGTH TRAINING (FULL BODY)

Resistance Band Exercises
Duration: 3 sets of 12 reps for each exercise.
How to Perform: Use resistance bands for exercises such as chest presses, rows, and leg extensions. Anchor the band securely and perform movements in a controlled manner.

DAY 11: REST DAY

DAY 10: FLEXIBILITY AND BALANCE

Stretching Routine
Duration: 30 minutes
How to Perform: Perform static stretches targeting major muscle groups, such as hamstrings, quadriceps, and shoulders. Hold each stretch for 20-30 seconds.

DAY 12: CARDIOVASCULAR EXERCISE

Light Jogging or Fast Walking
Duration: 30 minutes
How to Perform: Alternate between light jogging and brisk walking if jogging feels too strenuous. Maintain a steady pace and focus on proper breathing.

DAY 13: STRENGTH TRAINING (CORE)

Abdominal Exercises
Duration: 3 sets of 12 reps
How to Perform: Perform exercises such as seated crunches and leg lifts. Focus on controlled movements and proper alignment.

DAY 14: REST DAY

DAY 15: CARDIOVASCULAR EXERCISE

Rowing Machine
Duration: 30 minutes
How to Perform: Use a rowing machine with proper technique, focusing on engaging both the upper and lower body. Maintain a steady pace.

DAY 16: STRENGTH TRAINING (UPPER BODY)

Modified Push-Ups
Duration: 3 sets of 10 reps
How to Perform: Perform push-ups with knees on the ground if full push-ups are too challenging. Keep elbows at a 45-degree angle and lower your body until chest nearly touches the floor.

DAY 17: FLEXIBILITY AND BALANCE

Tai Chi
Duration: 30 minutes
How to Perform: Follow a Tai Chi routine focusing on slow, deliberate movements. This practice helps improve balance and flexibility.

DAY 18: REST DAY

DAY 19: CARDIOVASCULAR EXERCISE

Hiking on a Moderate Trail
Duration: 30 minutes
How to Perform: Choose a trail with a gentle incline. Wear appropriate footwear and pace yourself to maintain steady breathing.

DAY 20: STRENGTH TRAINING (LOWER BODY)

Standing Calf Raises
Duration: 3 sets of 15 reps
How to Perform: Once you have your feet hip-width apart, stand up and rise onto your toes. After that, lower yourself back down. In order to maintain your balance, you can use a chair or a wall.

DAY 21: REST DAY

DAY 22: CARDIOVASCULAR EXERCISE

Elliptical Trainer
Duration: 30 minutes
How to Perform: Use an elliptical trainer with a smooth, consistent motion. Adjust resistance and incline to match your fitness level.

DAY 23: STRENGTH TRAINING (FULL BODY)

Bodyweight Exercises
Duration: 3 sets of 10 reps for each exercise
How to Perform: Incorporate exercises like wall   sits, step-ups, and bodyweight lunges. Ensure proper form and gradual progression.

DAY 24: FLEXIBILITY AND BALANCE

Pilates
Duration: 30 minutes
How to Perform: Engage in Pilates exercises focusing on core strength, flexibility, and balance. Use a mat and follow a guided routine if available.

DAY 25: REST DAY

DAY 26: CARDIOVASCULAR EXERCISE

Dancing
Duration: 30 minutes
How to Perform: Dance to your favorite music at a comfortable pace. Enjoy the activity and focus on maintaining a consistent rhythm.

DAY 27: STRENGTH TRAINING (CORE AND FLEXIBILITY)

Planks and Side Planks
Duration: 3 sets of 30 seconds each
How to Perform: Assume a plank position on your elbows and toes, maintaining a straight line with your body throughout the exercise. Transition to side planks, holding all sides for the same duration.

DAY 28: REST DAY

5.4 Low-Impact Exercise for Men Over 60 Practicing Intermittent Fasting

Low-impact exercises are ideal for men over 60, especially those practicing intermittent fasting, as they reduce stress on the joints while still providing essential cardiovascular, strength, and flexibility benefits. These exercises are particularly beneficial for maintaining mobility, improving balance, and supporting overall well-being. Here's a comprehensive guide to incorporating low-impact exercises into your routine:

1. Walking

- **Benefits:** Improves cardiovascular health, aids weight management, and enhances overall endurance.

- **How to Perform:** Aim for brisk walking sessions of 30-45 minutes, 3-5 times per week. Choose a flat or gently inclined path, and maintain a pace that elevates your heart rate but still allows you to converse comfortably. Use supportive footwear and walk with good posture.

2. Swimming

- **Benefits**: Provides a full-body workout, reduces joint stress, and improves cardiovascular and muscular endurance.

- **How to Perform**: Swim laps or participate in water aerobics for 30 minutes, 2-3 times per week. The buoyancy of the water supports your body and minimizes impact on the joints. Focus on smooth, controlled movements to maximize the exercise's benefits.

3. Cycling

- **Benefits**: Enhances cardiovascular fitness, strengthens leg muscles, and is easy on the joints.

- **How to Perform**: Use a stationary bike or a regular bicycle. Your goal should be to cycle for 30 minutes at an even pace three to four times a week. Adjust the seat height for proper leg extension and maintain a steady cadence.

4. Chair Exercises

- **Benefits**: Suitable for those with limited mobility, helps strengthen muscles and improve flexibility.

- **How to Perform**: Perform seated exercises like seated marches, seated leg lifts, and seated torso twists. Aim for 15-20 minutes of exercise, 2-3 times per week. Use a sturdy chair with back support and ensure proper form.

5. Yoga

- **Benefits**: Improves flexibility, balance, and core strength while reducing stress.

■ **How to Perform**: Engage in a gentle yoga routine that includes poses such as Cat-Cow, Warrior I, and Tree Pose. Aim for 20-30 minutes of yoga, 2-3 times per week. Focus on slow, controlled movements and deep breathing. Consider a class designed for seniors or follow an online video for guidance.

6. Tai Chi

■ **Benefits**: Enhances balance, coordination, and mental relaxation through slow, flowing movements.

■ **How to Perform**: Participate in a Tai Chi class or follow a guided video. Practice for 20-30 minutes, 2-3 times per week. Focus on smooth, deliberate movements and maintaining a steady, relaxed pace.

7. Resistance Band Exercises

■ **Benefits**: Builds muscle strength and improves joint stability without heavy weights.

■ **How to Perform**: When performing exercises like bicep curls, chest presses, and leg extensions, resistance bands are an excellent tool to use. For each exercise, perform two to three sets of ten to twelve repetitions, two to three times a week. Adjust the band's resistance to match your strength level and ensure controlled movements.

8. Stretching

■ **Benefits**: Increases flexibility, reduces muscle tension, and improves range of motion.

■ **How to Perform**: Include in your regimen a stretching routine that focuses on important muscular groups, such as the hamstrings, quadriceps, shoulders, and back. Each stretch should be held for 20 to 30 seconds and then repeated two to three times. Perform stretching exercises daily or as part of your warm-up or cool-down routine.

Chapter 6: Breakfast Recipes For Intermittent Fasting

1. Power Protein Smoothie

This smoothie combines nutrient-rich ingredients like spinach, flaxseeds, and peanut butter, offering a balance of protein, healthy fats, and fiber to help maintain muscle mass and promote cardiovascular health. The inclusion of Greek yogurt provides a good source of probiotics, which support digestive health—an important aspect of overall wellness as we age. The healthy fats from peanut butter and flaxseeds help with satiety and hormone regulation, while the potassium-rich banana supports heart health and muscle function.

(Ready in: 5 minutes | Cook Duration: None | Persons: 2)

Necessary Items:

- Frozen spinach: 1 cup
- Ripe banana: 1
- Unsweetened almond milk or low-fat milk: 1 cup
- Plain Greek yogurt: 1/2 cup
- Ground flaxseeds: 1 tbsp
- Unsweetened peanut butter: 1 tbsp
- Protein powder (elective, based on preference): 1 scoop
- Ice cubes (elective, to adjust consistency): 1 cup

How to Prepare. Start by peeling the ripe banana. The components should be blended together in a mixer: spinach, banana, milk, Greek yogurt, ground flaxseeds, peanut butter, and protein powder if using. If you would like the consistency to be more substantial, you can include ice cubes in the mixer. Blend the components until they are completely smooth and properly blended. Modify the consistency by including a little bit more milk if it is too dense. Taste the smoothie and adjust to your preference. Once ready, pour into glasses and present instantly.

Nutritional Info (per serving, without elective honey/maple syrup and ice cubes):
Calories: 250 kcal, Protein: 13g, Carbohydrates: 30g, Fat: 10g, Saturated Fat: 1.5g, Cholesterol: 5mg, Sodium: 70mg, Potassium: 800mg, Sugars: 15g

2. High-Protein Pancakes

Designed to support muscle maintenance and recovery, these pancakes are rich in high-quality protein from both almond flour and whey protein powder. The inclusion of almond flour also provides healthy fats and fiber, which help regulate blood sugar levels and promote cardiovascular health—key concerns as men age. The applesauce adds natural sweetness without the need for added sugars, making these pancakes low in carbohydrates but still flavorful. Additionally, the healthy fats from the coconut oil contribute to heart health, while the eggs provide a complete protein source, essential for maintaining muscle mass.

(Ready in: 30 minutes | Cook Duration: 25 minutes | Persons: 2)

Necessary Items:

- 1/2 cup almond flour
- 1/4 cup whey protein powder (unflavored

- or vanilla)
- 1/2 tsp baking powder
- 1 tbsp unsweetened applesauce
- 2/3 tsp melted coconut oil
- 1/4 tsp salt1/2 cup unsweetened almond milk
- 1/2 tsp vanilla extract
- 2 big eggs

How to Prepare: Components such as almond flour, whey protein powder, baking powder, and salt should be mixed together in a big mixing dish. You should blend the almond milk, applesauce, melted coconut oil, vanilla extract, and eggs in another bowl and whisk them together until they are thoroughly blended. Start by making a well in the middle of the dry components, and then pour the liquid mixture into the well. Whisk the batter softly until it is almost completely incorporated; avoid overmixing. Allow the batter to rest for 10 to 15 minutes, which helps create fluffier pancakes by allowing the baking powder to activate. Preheating a non-stick skillet or frypan at a middling temp. and mildly coating it with cooking spray or a little quantity of coconut oil is the first step in the process. About a quarter cup of batter should be poured onto the pan for each individual pancake. Allow to cook for 2 to 3 minutes, or until bubbles appear on the surface and the edges have become firm. Cook the pancakes for a further 2 to 3 minutes after flipping them, until they have a golden brown color and are cooked all the way through. Repeat with the remaining batter, reapplying cooking spray or oil as needed.

Nutritional Info: Calories: 220kcal, Protein: 16g, Carbohydrates: 8g, Fiber: 3g, Sugars: 2g, Fat: 15g, Saturated Fat: 4.5g, Cholesterol: 160mg, Sodium: 210mg, Potassium: 150mg

3. Egg and Avocado on Sweet Potato Toast with Sautéed Kale

For men over 60 practicing intermittent fasting, this dish is an excellent balance of protein, healthy fats, and fiber, keeping you full and satisfied during your eating window. Sweet potatoes provide a slow-release carbohydrate, ideal for sustained energy, while kale and avocado offer powerful antioxidants and heart-healthy nutrients. This combination supports muscle function, cardiovascular health, and overall vitality, making it a perfect meal for healthy aging.

(Ready in: 20 minutes | Serves: 2)

Ingredients:

- 1 big sweet potato (sliced lengthwise into 1/2 inch dense slices)
- 2 eggs
- 1 ripe avocado
- 1 tsp lemon juice
- 2 tsps olive oil
- 1 cup fresh kale leaves (stems taken out, roughly severed)
- 1/4 cup crumbled feta cheese (elective)
- Salt & freshly ground black pepper (as needed)
- Red pepper flakes (elective for a kick)

Instructions: Warm up the oven to 400 deg.F (200 deg.C). To season the sweet potato slices, lightly spray them with olive oil and then season them with salt and pepper. After placing the slices on a baking sheet, bake them for 15 to 20 minutes, turning them over midway through the cooking process, until they are tender and mildly crispy on the edges. While the sweet potatoes are baking, cook the eggs to your liking (poached, fried, or soft-boiled).

The avocado should be mashed with lemon juice, salt, and pepper in a small bowl until it reaches a creamy consistency. Using a pan, bring 1 tsp of olive oil at a middling temp. Continue to sauté the severed kale for two to three minutes, or until it has become wilted and soft. The dish can be seasoned with salt, pepper, and, if preferred, a pinch of crushed red pepper flakes. When the sweet potato slices are finished cooking, include the mashed avocado to all slices and spread it evenly. Top with sautéed kale, then put the eggs on top. Sprinkle with crumbled feta cheese for extra flavor, if using. Present instantly.

Nutritional Info: Calories: 350 kcal , Protein: 12g, Carbohydrates: 35g, Fat: 20g, Fiber: 9g, Sugars: 7g, Sodium: 300mg, Potassium: 900mg

4. Sweet Potato and Turkey Breakfast Burritos

With a balance of complex carbohydrates, protein, and healthy fats, this meal supports sustained energy levels throughout the day. The inclusion of bell peppers and sweet potatoes adds a boost of vitamins A and C, which promote immune health and vision, while lean turkey provides muscle-supporting protein.

(Ready in: 35 minutes | Cook Duration: 25 minutes | Persons: 2)

Necessary Items:

- 4 whole wheat tortillas
- 1 medium sweet potato, skinned and cubed
- 1/2 lb. ground turkey
- 1/2 red bell pepper, severed
- 1/2 green bell pepper, severed
- 3 eggs, lightly beaten
- 1/4 cup shredded mozzarella cheese
- 1 tsp olive oil
- 1 tsp smoked paprika
- Salt and freshly ground black pepper (as needed)
- 1/4 cup fresh salsa (elective, for presenting)

How to Prepare: 1 tsp of olive oil should be heated in a big skillet to a middling temp. After including the sweet potato that has been cubed, flavor it with salt, pepper, and smoked paprika, and then cook it for 10 to 12 minutes while mixing it irregularly until it is soft and has a light-brown-colored appearance. The sweet potatoes should be moved to the side of the skillet, and then the ground turkey and sliced bell peppers should be added to the skillet. It is important to break apart the turkey while it cooks so that it may be browned and cooked all the way through. Mix the sweet potatoes with the other ingredients and whisk until everything is well incorporated. Put away for later. Scramble the eggs in a distinct pan with a little bit of oil until they are almost completely set. Take the pan off the heat and put it away. Warm the tortillas by wrapping them in aluminum foil and placing them in an oven that has been warmed up to 350 deg.F (175 deg.C) for 5 to 7 minutes. Lay each warm tortilla flat and fill with a portion of the sweet potato and turkey mixture, scrambled eggs, and a sprinkle of shredded mozzarella cheese. Roll the tortillas into burritos, tucking in the sides as you roll. Present the burritos with fresh salsa on the side if desired. Enjoy immediately.

Nutritional Info: Calories: 460kcal, Protein: 30g, Carbohydrates: 42g, Fiber: 7g, Sugars: 6g, Fat: 19g, Saturated Fat: 5g, Cholesterol: 220mg, Sodium: 750mg, Potassium: 850mg

5. High-Fiber Banana Nut Porridge

The combination of oats, flaxseeds, and banana provides a rich source of dietary fiber, which aids in digestion and supports cardiovascular health. Almond butter and walnuts include healthy fats and protein, promoting sustained energy and muscle maintenance. With natural sweetness from the banana and a boost of antioxidants from elective berries, this porridge is a delicious, nutrient-dense meal that fits seamlessly into your fasting regimen while supporting overall well-being.

(Ready in: 10 minutes | Cook Duration: 7 minutes | Persons: 3)

Necessary Items:

- 50g rolled oats
- 130ml water or unsweetened almond milk
- 1 ripe banana, cut
- 1 tbsp flaxseeds
- 1 tbsp almond butter
- 1 tsp cinnamon
- 1 pinch of salt
- 1 tbsp severed walnuts (elective, for garnish)
- Fresh berries (elective, for garnish)

How to Prepare: Using a small saucepan, bring the water or almond milk to a boil. Prepare the mixture. Include the rolled oats and a little bit of salt in the liquid that is now boiling. Lower the temp. to a low setting and let the porridge simmer for 5 to 7 minutes, mixing it irregularly until the oats have become tender and the consistency of the porridge has reached the appropriate level. Once the oats are cooked, stir in the sliced banana, flaxseeds, cinnamon, and almond butter. Mix well until the banana melts into the porridge, creating a naturally sweet and creamy texture. Divide the porridge into bowls. Garnish with severed walnuts and fresh berries, if desired. Present instantly for a warm, comforting breakfast.

Nutritional Info: Calories: 180kcal, Protein: 5g, Carbohydrates: 27g, Dietary Fiber: 6g, Sugars: 8g, Fat: 7g, Saturated Fat: 0.5g, Sodium: 55mg, Potassium: 300mg

6. Honey Almond Quinoa Granola

With a base of oats, puffed quinoa, and almonds, this granola delivers a combination of complex carbohydrates, healthy fats, and plant-based protein to keep you energized throughout the day. The chia seeds and sunflower seeds include extra fiber and omega-3 fatty acids, promoting heart health and digestion, while honey and dried apricots provide natural sweetness without excessive sugar.

(Ready in: 2 hrs 10 mins | Serves: 12 | Yield: 12 1/2 cup servings)

Ingredients:

- 1/2 cup sliced almonds
- 2 cups old-fashioned oats
- 1/2 cup puffed quinoa
- 1/4 cup chia seeds (for added fiber and omega-3)
- 1/4 tsp salt

- 1/4 cup raw honey
- 1 tbsp vanilla extract
- 1/4 cup coconut oil or 1/4 cup olive oil
- 1/4 cup sunflower seeds (elective, for added crunch)
- 1/4 cup dried apricots, severed (elective, for added sweetness)

Instructions: Using parchment paper, line a big baking sheet with a rim and warm up your oven to 200 deg.F (93 deg.C). Gather the oats, puffed quinoa, sliced almonds, chia seeds, and sunflower seeds (if you are using them) into a big bowl and mix them together. Honey, coconut oil (or olive oil), and salt should be mixed together in a small saucepan at a middling temp. until the honey is melted and thoroughly blended until the honey is completely dissolved. Take the pan off the heat and include the vanilla essence while stirring. To ensure every one of the dry components are thoroughly covered, pour the honey-oil mixture over them and whisk until everything is evenly distributed. Put the mixture in a uniform layer on the baking sheet that has been prepared. Bake the granola for approximately 2 hours without mixing it, or until it reaches golden-brown color and a crunchy texture. The granola should be taken out from the oven and allowed to cool entirely on the baking sheet before being taken out. Once cooled, stir in the severed dried apricots, if using. Break the granola into chunks before storing in a sealed container.

Nutritional Info: Calories: 210kcal, Protein: 6g, Carbohydrates: 23g, Fat: 6g, Fiber: 6g, Sugars: 8g, Saturated Fat: 2g, Sodium: 35mg, Potassium: 160mg

7. Savory Lentil & Veggie Scramble

This dish offers a protein-packed and nutrient-dense meal option for men over 60 practicing intermittent fasting. Lentils provide plant-based protein and fiber, while the addition of colorful vegetables adds vitamins and antioxidants. This dish helps sustain energy levels throughout the day without being too heavy, making it ideal for those who want a satisfying but healthy meal.

(Ready in: 15 minutes | Cook Duration: 15 minutes | Persons: 2)

Necessary Items:

- 1 can (15 oz) lentils, drained and washed
- 1 small zucchini, cubed
- 1 small carrot, grated
- 1/2 medium red onion, finely severed
- 1 piece garlic, crushed
- 1/2 tsp ground coriander
- 1/2 tsp smoked paprika
- 1/4 tsp ground turmeric
- 1/4 tsp chili flakes (elective, for a bit of heat)
- Salt and black pepper as needed
- 2 tbsps olive oil
- Fresh parsley or green onions for garnish (elective)

How to Prepare: After draining and washing the lentils, lay them aside for later use. At middling temp., bring the olive oil to a simmer in a big skillet. Sauté the red onion that has been severed and the garlic that has been crushed for around 2 to 3 minutes, or until the onion becomes translucent and fragrant. Toss in the cubed zucchini and grated carrot, cooking for further 3-4 minutes until the vegetables begin to soften. Sprinkle the ground coriander, smoked paprika, turmeric, and chili flakes into the skillet. Coat the vegetables with the spices by stirring them thoroughly. While mixing, include the lentils in the pan and make sure everything is thoroughly blended. Allow the flavors to blend for a further 5 to 7 minutes while the food is cooking. Include salt and pepper as needed and flavor with salt. Once the scramble is heated through and well-mixed, garnish with fresh parsley or severed green onions for a burst of freshness. Present instantly as a hearty breakfast, lunch, or dinner option.

Nutritional Info: Calories: 310kcal, Protein: 14g, Carbohydrates: 38g, Dietary Fiber: 12g, Sugars: 7g, Fat: 10g, Saturated Fat: 1.5g, Sodium: 480mg, Potassium: 640mg

---

8. Apple Cinnamon Almond Scones

These scones offer a warm and comforting breakfast option for men over 60 practicing intermittent fasting. The combination of apples, almonds, and cinnamon provides a rich source of antioxidants, fiber, and heart-healthy fats, making these scones a nutritious indulgence.

(Ready in: 15 minutes | Cook Duration: 15-18 min | Persons: 8 scones)

Necessary Items:

- 2 cups all-purpose flour
- 1/4 cup granulated sugar
- 2 1/2 tsps baking powder
- 1/2 tsp salt
- 1/2 cup unsalted butter, cold and cubed
- 1/2 cup finely severed almonds
- 1 medium apple, skinned and cubed
- 1/2 tsp ground cinnamon
- 1/2 cup whole or 2% milk
- 1 big egg
- 1 tsp vanilla extract
- Sugar for sprinkling on top (elective)

How to Prepare: Set your oven to 400 deg.F (200 deg.C). Make sure to put away a baking sheet that has been covered with parchment paper. Put the all-purpose flour, sugar, baking powder, salt, and ground cinnamon in a big mixing basin and whisk them together until they are blended. The dry base for your scones is created as a result of this. The chilled butter that has been cut into cubes should be added to the dry components. Work the butter into the flour with your fingers or a pastry cutter until the mixture forms coarse crumbs. This should take several minutes. The butter should still be in small chunks, which will help create a flaky texture in the scones. Gently fold in the finely severed almonds and cubed apple pieces, making sure that they are dispersed uniformly throughout the mixture. To make the vanilla extract, mix the milk, egg, and vanilla extract together in a separate basin. A soft dough should be formed by pouring the liquid mixture into the dry components and stirring it gently until it is combined.

Take care not to overmix the batter, as doing so can cause the scones to become rough. Put the dough on a surface that has been mildly dusted with flour and knead it a few times in a gentle manner. Form it into a disc that is circular and approximately one inch dense. Make eight wedges out of the dough by cutting it with a sharp knife or a bench scraper, and then put them on the baking sheet that has been prepared. For an additional layer of sweetness and crunch, you can sprinkle a little sugar on top of each scone if you so wish. As soon as the oven has been prepared, put the scones inside and bake them for 15 to 18 minutes, or until they have a golden-brown color and a toothpick that has been pushed into the center comes out clean. On a wire rack, the scones should be allowed to cool down a little before being served. It is recommended that you consume these scones while they are still warm; however, they can be refrigerated in a sealed container for up to 2 days.

Nutritional Info: Calories: 315kcal, Protein: 6g, Carbohydrates: 35g, Dietary Fiber: 3g, Sugars: 12g, Fat: 16g, Saturated Fat: 7g, Cholesterol: 50mg, Sodium: 350mg, Potassium: 190mg

9. Banana Walnut Oatmeal

This dish provides a balanced combination of complex carbohydrates, fiber, and healthy fats, offering sustained energy throughout the day. The oats and bananas are rich in soluble fiber, which supports heart health and aids digestion, while walnuts contribute omega-3 fatty acids that promote brain function and decrease inflammation. The moderate amount of natural sugars from bananas and honey helps curb cravings without spiking blood sugar levels.

(Ready in: 5 minutes | Cook Duration: 10 minutes | Persons: 2)

Necessary Items:

- 1 cup old-fashioned rolled oats
- 2 cups milk (dairy or a non-dairy alternative such as almond or oat milk)
- 1 medium ripe banana, mashed
- 1 tbsp honey or maple syrup (adjust for sweetness)
- 1 tsp cinnamon
- 1/4 tsp salt
- 1/4 cup severed walnuts (elective, for topping)
- 1 tbsp chia seeds (elective, for added fiber and omega-3s)
- Additional honey or maple syrup for drizzling (elective)

How to Prepare: The rolled oats and milk should be mixed together in a saucepan of medium size. The mashed banana, honey or maple syrup, cinnamon, and salt should be stirred in at this point. Make sure every one of the components are thoroughly mixed together. The mixture should be brought to a boil at a middling temp. in the saucepan, and then bring it to a simmer. Once boiling, decrease the temp. to low and let it simmer for 7-10 minutes, mixing irregularly, until the oatmeal reaches your desired creamy consistency. The oats should be split between two dishes once it has been cooked. Top with severed walnuts for a crunchy texture and chia seeds for added nutrition. If you like, drizzle a bit more honey or maple syrup on top for extra sweetness.

Nutritional Info: Calories: 310kcal, Protein: 10g, Carbohydrates: 52g, Dietary Fiber: 8g, Sugars: 15g, Fat: 8g, Saturated Fat: 1g, Cholesterol: 10mg, Sodium: 320mg, Potassium: 400mg

10. Blueberry Almond Muffins

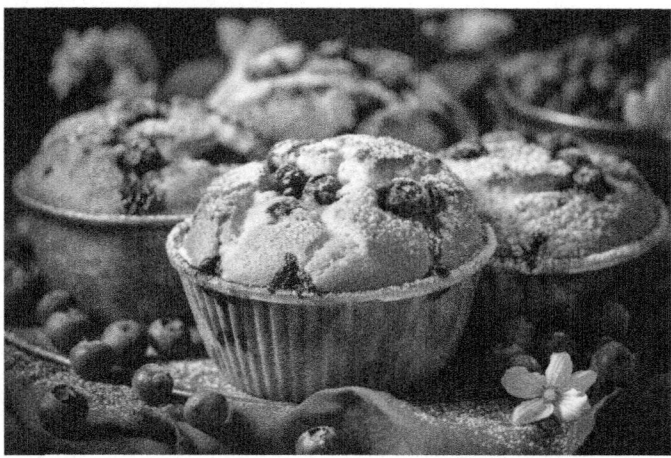

These muffins are packed with antioxidants, fiber, and healthy fats, making them a great choice for men over 60 who are following an intermittent fasting regime. Blueberries support heart health and cognitive function, both crucial as we age. Almond flour adds healthy fats and protein, keeping you full for longer, while the whole wheat flour provides essential fiber.

(Preparation Time: 45 minutes | Servings: 12)

Ingredients:

- 2 cups whole wheat flour
- 1 cup almond flour
- 1/2 cup coconut sugar or brown sugar
- 1 tsp baking powder
- 1 tsp baking soda
- 1/4 tsp salt
- 1 1/2 cups fresh or frozen blueberries
- 1/4 cup olive oil or avocado oil
- 1 cup unsweetened almond milk (or any dairy-free alternative)
- 1 tsp vanilla extract
- 1/2 tsp ground cinnamon (elective)
- 1/4 cup severed almonds (elective, for topping)

Instructions: Prepare a muffin tin with a capacity of 12 cups by mildly greasing it or covering it with muffin liners and preheating the oven to 350 deg.F (180 deg.C). To ensure that the components are thoroughly mixed together, put the whole wheat flour, almond flour, coconut sugar, baking powder, baking soda, cinnamon (if using), and salt in a large basin and whisk them together. An olive oil, almond milk, and vanilla extract mixture should be mixed together in a distinct basin until it is completely smooth. Pour the liquid mixture into the bowl containing the dry components in a slow and steady manner. Gradually stir until the components are almost completely mixed. Blueberries should be folded in carefully, making sure that they are distributed evenly. Spread the batter out evenly among the wells of the muffin tin that has been prepared. In order to give some texture to the tops, you might choose to sprinkle them with severed almonds.

In an oven that has been warmed up, the muffin pan should be put, and the muffins should be baked for 25 to 30 minutes, or until the tops of the muffins have a golden brown color and a toothpick that has been immersed into the center of the muffins remains clean. The muffins should be allowed to cool for around 10 to 15 minutes in the muffin tray before being transferred to a wire rack to finish cooling altogether. Warm up and enjoy, or put away for later. **Chef's Tip:** You can freeze these muffins for up to a month. Wrap them individually in plastic wrap or foil before placing them in a sealed container or resealable freezer bag. To thaw, leave them overnight in the fridge or microwave them for 20 to 30 seconds.

Nutritional Info: Calories: 210 kcal, Protein: 5g, Carbohydrates: 28g, Dietary Fiber: 5g, Sugars: 10g, Fat: 9g, Saturated Fat: 1g, Sodium: 150mg, Potassium: 180mg

11. Egg Scramble with Sweet Potatoes
(Preparation Time: 10 minutes | Cooking Time: 20 minutes | Servings: 2)

Ingredients:

- 1/2 cup severed onion
- 1 (8-oz) sweet potato, cubed
- 2 tsps severed rosemary
- Salt, as needed
- 4 big eggs
- 4 big egg whites
- Pepper, as needed
- 2 tbsps severed chives

Instructions: Warm up the oven to 425 deg.F (220 deg.C). Mix the sweet potato cubes, onion that has been cut into pieces, rosemary that has been cut into pieces, salt, and pepper in a baking dish. Spray the sweet potatoes with cooking spray and roast them for around 20 minutes, or until they reach the desired tenderness. In a bowl of medium size, blend the eggs, egg whites, and a pinch of salt and pepper by whisking them together. The eggs should be scrambled for approximately 5 minutes at middling temp. in a skillet that has been sprayed with cooking spray. Present the scrambled eggs with the roasted sweet potatoes and sprinkle with severed chives.

Nutritional Info: Calories: 571, Protein: 44g, Carbohydrates: 52g (including 9g of fiber). Fat: 20g

12. Sunflower Seed Butter Apple Toast
This quick and nutritious meal is perfect for breaking your fast, offering a balanced intake of macronutrients to support healthy aging. Whole-grain or sprouted bread provides a good source of complex carbohydrates, while sunflower seed butter delivers healthy fats and protein, which help in maintaining muscle mass and energy levels. The fiber-rich apple slices, paired with flax seeds, support digestion and heart health, which are critical for aging men. The addition of pomegranate seeds or other fruits boosts antioxidants, helping to reduce inflammation and promote longevity.

(Ready in: 5 minutes | Cook Duration: 5 minutes | Persons: 2)

Necessary Items:

- Bread, whole-grain or sprouted: 4 slices
- Sunflower seed butter (or your preferred seed butter): 2 tbsps
- Cinnamon, ground: 1 tsp
- Apple, finely cut: 1 medium
- Flax seeds (elective, for added omega-3 and fiber): 1 tbsp
- Maple syrup (elective, for a light drizzle): 2 tbsps
- Pomegranate seeds or other fresh fruit (elective, for garnish)

How to Prepare: Toast your slices of whole-grain or sprouted bread until golden and crispy. Disperse a fine layer of sunflower seed butter evenly on each slice. Arrange the thin apple slices over the seed butter, ensuring even coverage. Sprinkle ground cinnamon on top of the apple slices to your taste. Optionally, sprinkle flax seeds evenly over the slices for added texture and nutrition. If desired, drizzle a touch of maple syrup over the top for a subtle sweetness. Garnish with pomegranate seeds or other fresh fruit for a burst of color and flavor.

Nutritional Info: Calories: 210kcal, Protein: 6g, Carbohydrates: 28g, Dietary Fiber: 5g, Sugars: 8g, Fat: 9g, Saturated Fat: 1g, Cholesterol: 0mg, Sodium: 160mg, Potassium: 270mg

13. Egg and Cheese Quesadilla

This satisfying meal helps maintain muscle mass and energy levels post-fasting, supporting overall health during the aging process. Eggs are rich in high-quality protein and essential nutrients like vitamin D and choline, which support muscle maintenance and brain health—key areas of focus for aging men. The whole-wheat tortillas provide complex carbohydrates that offer sustained energy, while the mix of bell peppers, onions, and tomatoes adds a variety of antioxidants to combat inflammation. Cheddar cheese contributes calcium for bone health, and the healthy fats from olive oil promote heart wellness.

(Ready in: 10 minutes | Cook Duration: 10 minutes | Persons: 2)

Necessary Items:

- Eggs, big: 4
- Milk: 1/4 cup
- Flavor as per your preference with salt and pepper
- Tortillas, whole-wheat and small: 4
- Cheddar cheese, shredded: 1 cup
- Bell peppers, cubed (be it red, green, or a mix): 1/2 cup
- Onions, finely cubed: 1/2 cup
- Tomatoes, cubed: 1/2 cup
- Olive oil: 2 tbsps
- Cilantro leaves, fresh (a delightful elective garnish)

How to Prepare: In a preferred mixing bowl, whisk together eggs, milk, salt, and pepper. Ensure each ingredient is seamlessly integrated for a unified blend. Spread out your tortillas, each primed to embrace an array of flavors. Garnish two tortillas generously with shredded cheddar, setting the stage for their delicious counterparts. In a skillet at middling temp., warm a drizzle of olive oil. Once heated, introduce bell peppers and onions, sautéing until they soften, typically 3-4 minutes. Towards the end, fold in the cubed tomatoes, allowing them to meld for further 1-2 minutes.

Blend your previously blended eggs with the sautéed vegetables in the skillet. Gently scramble until the eggs are soft and fully integrated with the veggies. Onto your cheese-laden tortillas, spread the scrambled egg mixture evenly. Top with the remaining tortillas, forming a delightful layered medley. Clean your skillet briefly, then return it to medium heat. Carefully place each quesadilla into the skillet, cooking all sides for 2-3 minutes or until they attain a golden hue and the cheese is melt-in-your-mouth luscious. After a brief pause, deftly slice the quesadillas into halves or neat quarters. A scattering of freshly severed cilantro provides a vibrant garnish.

Nutritional Info: Calories: 380 kcal, Protein: 18g, Carb: 22g, Dietary Fiber: 3g, Sugars: 5g, Fat: 25g, Saturated Fat: 10g, Cholesterol: 299mg, Sodium: 488mg, Potassium: 297mg

14. Prune Walnut Energy Bites

Prunes are rich in antioxidants and fiber, which support digestive health and reduce inflammation—essential factors for healthy aging. Walnuts provide healthy omega-3 fats, which benefit heart and brain function. Chia seeds contribute extra fiber and plant-based protein, making these bites an excellent post-fasting snack to replenish energy and keep you feeling full longer. The natural sweetness of prunes and elective maple syrup makes this a delicious treat without refined sugar.

(Ready in: 15 minutes | Persons: 12 bites)

Necessary Items:

- Prunes, dried: 1 cup
- Walnuts: 1 cup
- Chia seeds: 1/4 cup

- Maple syrup (elective for natural sweetness): 1 tbsp
- Cinnamon (an elective flavor enhancer): 1/2 tsp
- A subtle hint of salt

How to Prepare: Ensure your prunes are pit-free, and all other ingredients are measured and ready. In a food processor, blend the dried prunes, walnuts, chia seeds, maple syrup (if using), cinnamon, and a pinch of salt. Pulse until the components form a sticky, cohesive mixture that holds together when pressed between your fingers. Scoop out small portions of the mixture with clean hands, shaping them into bite-sized balls or compact squares. After placing the energy bites in the fridge for approximately half an hour, they will become more solid. Once set, these bites are ready to be enjoyed. For convenient and nutritious snacks throughout the week, store any leftovers in a container that can be sealed and placed in a fridge.

Nutritional Info: Calories: 85 kcal, Protein: 2g, Carbohydrates: 11g, Dietary Fiber: 3g, Sugars: 8g, Fat: 4g, Saturated Fat: 0.5g, Cholesterol: 0mg, Sodium: 2mg, Potassium: 180mg

15. Chickpea and Carrot Spread Sandwich

This sandwich is an excellent choice for men over 60 following an intermittent fasting regimen due to its balance of fiber, plant-based protein, and healthy fats that help stabilize blood sugar levels and promote satiety. Carrots provide vitamin A for skin and eye health, while cucumber and alfalfa sprouts offer hydration and additional nutrients. Whole-grain bread delivers a steady release of complex carbohydrates, helping to maintain energy levels and support overall well-being during fasting periods.

(Ready in: 5 minutes | Persons: 1)

Necessary Items:

- Whole-grain bread: 2 slices
- Chickpea spread (hummus): 2 tbsps
- Carrots, grated: 1/2 cup
- Cucumber, finely cut: 4-6 slices
- Alfalfa sprouts (elective, for extra nutrients): A handful
- Lemon juice: A few drops
- Salt and pepper: As required

How to Prepare: Spread a generous layer of chickpea spread on one slice of whole-grain bread. Top with grated carrots to include a crunchy texture. Layer thin slices of cucumber for freshness. For additional nutrients, include a handful of alfalfa sprouts if desired. To include a bit of zest, drizzle a couple of drops of lemon juice over the dish. Include salt and pepper as needed and flavor with salt. The second slice of bread should be placed on top, and a little press should be applied. If desired, the sandwich can be sliced in two. Enjoy immediately.

Nutritional Info: Calories: 280kcal, Protein: 8g, Carbohydrates: 38g, Dietary Fiber: 9g, Sugars: 5g, Fat: 10g, Saturated Fat: 1.5g, Cholesterol: 0mg, Sodium: 270mg, Potassium: 600mg

16. Cottage Cheese and Veggie Lettuce Wraps

Low-fat cottage cheese provides high-quality protein to support muscle mass and satiety while keeping fat content in check. The fresh vegetables include fiber and essential vitamins, supporting digestive health and overall well-being. The use of apple cider vinegar offers a tangy flavor while potentially aiding in digestion and stabilizing blood sugar levels. The wrap is low in calories but rich in nutrients, making it an excellent choice for maintaining energy and health during eating windows.

(Prep Time: 10 minutes | Servings: 2)

Ingredients:

- 4 big lettuce leaves (e.g., romaine or butter lettuce)
- 1 cup low-fat cottage cheese
- 1/2 cucumber, finely cut
- 1/2 red bell pepper, finely cut
- 1/4 red onion, finely cut
- 1 tbsp severed fresh chives
- 2 tsps apple cider vinegar
- Salt and pepper as needed

Instructions: Arrange the lettuce leaves flat on a clean surface. Spread the cottage cheese evenly across the center of each lettuce leaf. Top with cucumber slices, red bell pepper slices, and red onion slices. Sprinkle with severed fresh chives and drizzle with apple cider vinegar. Include salt and pepper as needed, and flavor with salt. Wraps can be made by carefully rolling the lettuce leaves into a roll. Present immediately or wrap in parchment paper for a convenient on-the-go meal.

Nutritional Info: Cals: 140kcal | Carbohydrates: 9g | Protein: 11g | Fat: 6g | Saturated Fat: 2g | Cholesterol: 20mg | Sodium: 180mg | Fiber: 3g | Sugar: 4g | Calcium: 120mg | Iron: 1mg

17. Greek Yogurt with Apple and Almonds

This dish fits well within an intermittent fasting regimen, offering a balanced, nutritious option to break your fast while supporting muscle maintenance and digestive health. Greek yogurt provides a high-quality source of protein, which helps maintain muscle mass and promotes satiety. The apple adds natural sweetness and fiber, aiding in digestive health and providing sustained energy. Almonds contribute healthy fats and additional protein, supporting heart health and overall well-being.

(Ready in: 5 minutes | Persons: 2)

Necessary Items:

- 1 cup Greek yogurt (plain, non-fat or low-fat)
- 1 small apple, cubed
- 1 tbsp slivered almonds
- 1 tsp honey (elective, for added sweetness)
- A sprinkle of cinnamon (elective)

How to Prepare: Begin by dicing a crisp, fresh apple into small cubes. In a mixing bowl, blend the Greek yogurt with the cubed apple. If desired, include a drizzle of honey for a touch of sweetness. Sprinkle slivered almonds on top for a satisfying crunch and a boost of healthy fats. For added flavor, you can also sprinkle a touch of cinnamon. Gently stir to mix everything together, and present instantly.

Nutritional Info: Calories: 180 kcal, Protein: 22g, Carb: 15g, Dietary, Fiber: 4g, Sugars: 14g, Fat: 6g, Saturated Fat: 1g, Cholesterol: 10mg, Sodium: 70mg, Calcium: 150mg, Iron: 0,8mg

18. Blueberry Spinach Smoothie

This smoothie is easy to prepare and fits well into a fasting routine, offering a nutritious and refreshing option to break your fast. The smoothie provides a good balance of protein from Greek yogurt, which helps maintain muscle mass and aids in recovery. Blueberries offer antioxidants and vitamins, contributing to overall health and reducing inflammation. Both the heart and the digestive system can benefit from the presence of omega-3 fatty acids and fiber, which are both found in chia seeds. Spinach, while elective, adds additional vitamins and minerals.

(Ready in: 5 minutes | Persons: 2)

Necessary Items:

- 1 cup unsweetened almond milk
- 1 cup frozen blueberries
- 1/2 cup plain Greek yogurt (low-fat)
- 1 tbsp chia seeds
- 1 tbsp honey (elective, for added sweetness)
- A handful of ice cubes
- A small handful of fresh spinach leaves (elective, for added nutrients)

How to Prepare: Prepare your ingredients by gathering them together. In a mixer, blend the unsweetened almond milk with the frozen blueberries. Include the Greek yogurt for a creamy texture and a tbsp of chia seeds for an extra boost of omega-3s and fiber. If you prefer a touch of sweetness, drizzle in some honey. For added freshness, toss in a small handful of spinach leaves. If you want your smoothie to be colder, include a handful of ice cubes to the mixture. Make sure the lid is on the blender, and blend until the mixture is completely smooth and consistent. After pouring the smoothie into glasses, you can either have it right now or put it in the fridge to make a nutritious snack that you can enjoy quickly.

Nutritional Info: Calories: 180 kcal, Protein: 9g, Carbohydrates: 25g, Dietary, Fiber: 6g, Sugars: 17g, Fat: 4g, Saturated Fat: 0.5g, Cholesterol: 2mg, Sodium: 110mg, Potassium: 300mg

19. Quinoa Breakfast Bowl with Apple and Walnuts

This nutrient-rich breakfast is easy to digest, making it a suitable option to break your fast with sustained energy and balanced nutrition. This bowl offers a balance of protein from quinoa and chia seeds, which supports muscle maintenance and overall health. The addition of walnuts provides healthy fats and omega-3 fatty acids, favorable for heart health. Apples include fiber and vitamins, while the honey or maple syrup provides a touch of natural sweetness without excessive added sugars.

(Ready in: 10 minutes | Cook Duration: 15 minutes | Persons: 2)

Necessary Items:

- 1 cup quinoa
- 2 cups water
- 1 cup unsweetened almond milk (or milk of your choice)
- 2 tbsps honey or maple syrup
- 1 tsp vanilla extract
- 1 apple, cubed
- 1/4 cup walnuts, severed
- 2 tbsps chia seeds
- A pinch of cinnamon (elective)

How to Prepare: To begin, eliminate any lingering bitterness from the quinoa by washing it under cold water several times. Put the quinoa that has been washed into a pot along with two cups of water. After bringing it to a boil, decrease the temp. to a low setting and cover the pot. The quinoa should be allowed to simmer for around fifteen minutes, or until it has absorbed all of the water and is soft. Allow it to recuperate for a couple of minutes. The almond milk should be warmed up in another pot located at low temp.

Stir in the honey or maple syrup and vanilla extract. Mix until thoroughly blended and then take out from temp. After the quinoa has been cooked, split it between two bowls. Pour the warm almond milk mixture over the quinoa. Top with cubed apple, severed walnuts, and chia seeds. For added flavor, sprinkle a pinch of cinnamon if desired.

Nutritional Info: Calories: 370 kcal, Protein: 10g, Carbohydrates: 56g, Dietary Fiber: 9g, Sugars: 18g, Fat: 12g, Saturated Fat: 1g, Cholesterol: 0mg, Sodium: 60mg, Potassium: 450mg

20. Baked Pears with Almonds and Cinnamon

This recipe is tailored to provide a satisfying, nutrient-dense option that aligns with intermittent fasting routines. Pears are a good source of dietary fiber and vitamin C, which support digestion and immune health. Almonds include healthy fats and protein, which are essential for maintaining muscle mass and overall energy levels. The cinnamon and nutmeg not only enhance flavor but also offer antioxidant benefits. This dish is low in saturated fat and cholesterol, making it heart-healthy and ideal for maintaining cardiovascular health.

(Prep Time: 10 minutes | Cook Time: 30 minutes | Servings: 4)

Ingredients:

- 4 medium-sized pears (such as Bosc or Anjou)
- 1/4 cup sliced almonds
- 2 tbsps agave syrup or honey
- 1 tsp ground cinnamon
- 1/4 tsp ground nutmeg
- 1 tbsp melted coconut oil
- 1/2 cup water

Instructions: Set your oven to 375 deg.F (190 deg.C). Prepare a baking dish by lightly greasing it or covering it with parchment paper. Core the pears, ensuring to leave the bottoms intact to hold the filling. In a small bowl, blend sliced almonds, agave syrup or honey, ground cinnamon, ground nutmeg, and melted coconut oil. Mix well to create a sticky filling. Spoon the almond mixture into the center of each pear, packing it slightly. Put the pears upright in the baking dish. In order to assist in the process of steaming the pears, pour the water into the bottom of the baking dish. Ten minutes into the baking process, cover with aluminum foil and bake. When the pears have reached the desired level of tenderness and mild caramelization, take out the foil and continue baking for a further 10 minutes. Enjoy warm, optionally garnished with a sprinkle of extra cinnamon or a dollop of low-fat Greek yogurt.

Nutritional Info: Calories: 180 kcal | Carbohydrates: 32g | Protein: 3g | Fat:7g | Saturated Fat: 2g | Sodium: 5mg | Fiber: 6g | Sugar: 20g | Potassium: 240mg

Chapter 6: Lunch Recipes For Intermittent Fasting

1. Lemon Herb Salmon with Roasted Brussels Sprouts

The dish is low in sodium and cholesterol, making it heart-friendly and suitable for maintaining a balanced diet during your eating window. Salmon is an abundant source of very nutritious omega-3 fatty acids and high-quality protein, both of which are helpful to the health of the heart and the function of the brain. The inclusion of lemon and herbs provides a flavor boost without additional calories, while Brussels sprouts offer fiber, vitamins, and antioxidants, contributing to digestive health and overall well-being.

(Ready in: 10 mins | Cook Duration: 20 mins | Persons: 2)

Necessary Items:

- 2 salmon fillets
- 2 tbsps olive oil
- 1 tbsp lemon juice
- 1 tsp dried dill
- 1 tsp dried thyme
- 1/2 tsp garlic powder
- 1/2 tsp onion powder
- 2 cups Brussels sprouts, trimmed and divided
- Salt and black pepper, as needed
- Fresh parsley (elective, for garnish)
- Lemon wedges (for presenting)

How to Prepare: Prepare your oven to 400 deg.F (200 deg.C). Olive oil, lemon juice, dried dill, dried thyme, garlic powder, and onion powder should be combined in a small bowl so that they can be thoroughly combined. The salmon fillets should be coated with this mixture evenly. Use salt and black pepper to season the food. The Brussels sprouts should be divided and placed in a bowl with a small amount of olive oil, some salt, and some black pepper. On a baking sheet, arrange them in a single layer and spread them about. Arrange the salmon fillets and the Brussels sprouts on the same baking sheet using the same method. The salmon should be able to be readily flaked with a fork, and the Brussels sprouts should be soft and mildly caramelized. Bake for 15 to 20 minutes with the salmon. Garnish the salmon with fresh parsley if desired and present with lemon wedges for extra zest. Arrange the roasted Brussels sprouts alongside the salmon for a complete meal.

Nutritional Info: Calories: 330 kcal Protein: 28g, Carbohydrates: 15g, Dietary Fiber: 5g, Sugars: 6g, Fat: 17g, Saturated Fat: 3g, Cholesterol: 75mg, Sodium: 170mg, Potassium: 800mg

2. Grilled Eggplant and Spinach Panini

The dish is relatively low in sodium and cholesterol, making it heart-friendly and suitable for a balanced diet during your eating window. The eggplant provides a good source of dietary fiber and antioxidants, supporting digestive health and reducing inflammation. Spinach adds essential vitamins and minerals like iron and calcium, while the ricotta and mozzarella cheese offer high-quality protein for muscle maintenance. Consuming bread made with whole grains not only helps to keep blood sugar levels stable but also guarantees a consistent release of energy.

(Prep Time: 90 mins | Cook time: 20min Persons: 2)

Necessary Items:

- 2 tbsps severed fresh basil
- 2 tbsps olive oil
- 2 oz. ricotta cheese
- 1/2 medium eggplant, cut into 1/2-inch slices (about 6 slices)
- 1 ounce shredded mozzarella cheese

- 1 tbsp grated Parmesan cheese
- 1/2 tsp salt
- 1 cup marinara sauce (low-sodium)
- 1/2 cup fresh spinach leaves
- 2 whole-grain panini rolls or ciabatta bread

How to Prepare: After sprinkling the eggplant slices with salt, set them in a colander and allow them to drain for around half an hour to collect any extra moisture. Take out the salt from the slices, then dry them with paper towels after rinsing them. A grill pan and 1 tbsp of olive oil should be heated together at a middling temp. Grill all slices of eggplant for approximately 3 to 4 minutes on all sides, or until it is soft and has a light char. Put it away for later. Ricotta cheese, mozzarella cheese that has been shredded, grated Parmesan cheese, and severed basil should be mixed together in a medium basin. The whole-grain rolls or ciabatta bread should be cut in half for this recipe. A fine layer of marinara sauce should be spread on the inside of each roll. A few fresh spinach leaves should be placed on the bottom half of each roll, and then the grilled eggplant slices should be placed on top of that. The cheese mixture should be spread over the eggplant, and then the top half of the roll should be used after that. An application of the leftover olive oil should be made on the exterior of the bread. Prepare a grill pan or panini press by heating it over a medium flame. Cook the sandwiches on the grill for approximately 3 to 4 minutes on all sides, or until the cheese has melted and the bread has become crispy. To present the panini warm, cut it in half and present it.

Nutritional Info: Calories: 330kcal, Protein: 15g, Carb: 35g, Dietary Fiber: 8g, Sugars: 8g, Fat: 15g, Saturated Fat: 5g, Cholesterol: 30mg, Sodium: 500mg, Potassium: 600mg

3. Sweet Potato and Black Bean Burrito

A satisfying and nutritious option for men over 60 on intermittent fasting. Sweet potatoes offer vitamins and fiber, while black beans provide protein and additional fiber, supporting digestion and sustained energy. This meal helps stabilize blood sugar and supports heart health, making it a great choice for breaking your fast.

(Ready in: 1hr, 5mins | Serves: 1 burrito)

Ingredients:

- 2 cups skinned and cubed sweet potatoes
- 2 tsps vegetable oil or vegetable broth
- 1/2 tsp salt
- 1 and 1/2 cups cubed onions
- 1 tbsp crushed fresh green chili pepper
- 4 garlic pieces, crushed (or pressed)
- 4 tsps ground cumin
- 1/2 cup lightly packed cilantro leaves
- 1/2 tsp salt
- 1 can (15 oz.) black beans, drained and washed
- 1 tsp ground coriander
- 2 tbsps fresh lemon juice
- 12 (10 inches) flour tortillas
- Fresh salsa for topping

Instructions: Warm up oven to 175 deg.C (350 deg.F). Include the sweet potatoes that have been cut into cubes to a saucepan of medium size and just enough water to cover them. Incorporate a 1/2 tsp of salt. The sweet potatoes should be cooked for approximately 10 minutes, after which the heat should be reduced to a simmer and the mixture should be brought to a boil. Drain, then set aside for later use. In a skillet or saucepan of medium size, bring the vegetable broth or vegetable oil to a temperature of medium-low before proceeding. The green chilli pepper, crushed garlic, and sliced onions should be added at this point. Over the course of approximately 7 minutes, cover the pan and cook the onions while tossing them intermittently. Include the ground cumin and ground coriander in the mixture that contains the onions. Cook for a further 2 to 3 minutes while stirring the mixture regularly. Take the pan off the heat and put it away. Put the cooked sweet potatoes, black beans, fresh lemon juice, cilantro leaves, and a 1/2 tsp of salt into a food processor and pulse until everything is nicely combined. Blend the components in a big bowl and mash them by hand or blend them until they are completely smooth. The sweet potato and black bean mixture should be transferred to a big mixing bowl, and then the onion and spice mixture that has been cooked should be mixed in. A big baking dish should be lightly oiled. Place around 2/3 to 3/4 of a cup of the filling in the middle of each tortilla. Before placing the tortillas in the baking dish, roll them up and arrange them with the seam side down. Wrap the baking dish in aluminum foil and put it in the oven for 30 minutes or until the burritos have reached the desired temperature. Present the Sweet Potato and Black Bean Burritos with fresh salsa on top.

Nutritional Info: Calories: 353 kcal, Protein: 8g, Carbohydrates: 59g, Fat: 9g, Fiber: 10g, Sugar: 4g, Sodium: 654mg

4. Lemon Herb Chicken and Veggie Skewers

This Lemon Herb Chicken and Veggie Skewers recipe offers a balanced meal ideal for men over 60 on intermittent fasting. The lean chicken provides high-quality protein to support muscle health, while a variety of colorful vegetables deliver essential vitamins and antioxidants. The combination of lemon and herbs not only adds flavor but also contributes to heart health and aids in digestion.

(Ready in: 20 mins | Cook Duration: 15 mins | Persons: 4)

Necessary Items:

- Chicken breasts, boneless and skinless, cubed: 1 lb.
- Red bell pepper, chunked: 1
- Green bell pepper, chunked: 1
- Red onion, chunked: 1
- Mushrooms, whole or divided: 1 cup
- Cherry tomatoes: 8-10
- Lemon juice: 2 tbsps
- Olive oil: 1/4 cup
- Garlic, crushed: 2 pieces
- Dried basil: 1 tsp
- Dried rosemary: 1 tsp
- Salt and pepper: as needed
- Wooden skewers (soaked in water for 30 minutes)

How to Prepare: Blend lemon juice, olive oil, crushed garlic, basil, rosemary, salt, and pepper in a bowl. After including the chicken cubes, marinate them for 15 minutes. Toss bell peppers, onion, mushrooms, and cherry tomatoes with the remaining marinade. Thread marinated chicken and vegetables onto soaked skewers. Turn the grill up to a medium-high temp. If you want the chicken to be cooked and the vegetables to be tender, grill the skewers for 5 to 7 minutes on all sides.

Nutritional Info: Calories: 275 kcal, Protein: 25g, Carbohydrates: 10g, Dietary Fiber: 3g, Sugars: 6g, Fat: 15g, Saturated Fat: 2g, Cholesterol: 70mg, Sodium: 80mg, Potassium: 600mg

5. Lemon Basil Grilled Cod

This Lemon Basil Grilled Cod offers a lighter alternative rich in lean protein and healthy fats. The lemon and basil enhance flavor while providing antioxidants and digestive benefits. This easy-to-prepare dish supports muscle health and energy levels without overloading your system, making it a perfect addition to your balanced eating plan.

(Prep Time: 10 minutes | Cook Time: 12 minutes | Servings: 4)

Ingredients:

- 4 cod fillets (about 6 oz. each)
- 2 tbsps lemon zest
- 2 tbsps olive oil
- 2 tbsps fresh lemon juice
- 1 tbsp fresh basil, severed
- 2 pieces garlic, crushed
- Salt and pepper: as needed
- Lemon slices and fresh basil for garnish

Instructions: To form the dressing, blend the lemon zest, olive oil, lemon juice, severed basil, crushed garlic, and seasonings of your choice in a small bowl. After placing the cod fillets in a shallow dish, apply the marinade to them and coat them. Marinate for 10 minutes prior to presenting. Warm up the grill to medium-high. Oil the grill grates to avoid them from sticking. Cod fillets should be grilled for 4 to 5 minutes on all sides, or until the fish is opaque and easily flakes apart with a fork on contact. Take out from grill and garnish with lemon slices and fresh basil.

Nutritional Info: Calories: 300kcal | Protein: 32g | Fat: 15g | Saturated Fat: 3g | Cholesterol: 80mg | Sodium: 85mg | Carbohydrates: 2g | Fiber: 0g | Sugar: 0g

6. Lemon Garlic Shrimp Sauté

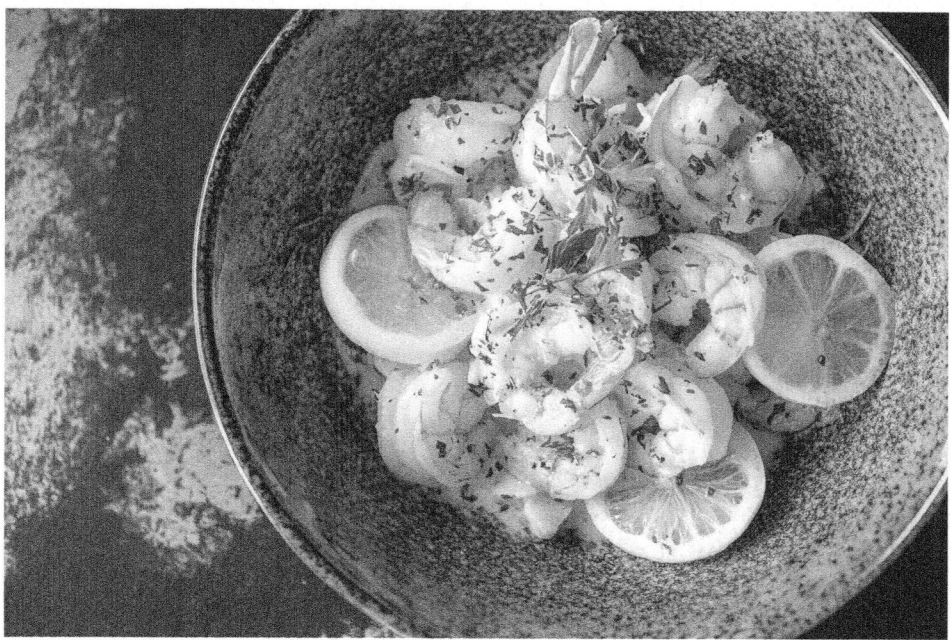

With its high protein content and minimal carbs, this dish perfect for supporting muscle health and maintaining satiety. The lemon and garlic offer antioxidants and digestive benefits, enhancing overall well-being while including a burst of fresh flavor.

(Ready in: 10 mins | Cook Duration: 8-10 mins | Persons: 4)

Necessary Items:

- 1 lb. big shrimp, skinned and deveined
- 2 tbsps olive oil
- 3 pieces garlic, crushed
- Zest of 1 lemon
- Juice of 1 lemon
- 1 tsp dried thyme
- 1/2 tsp smoked paprika
- Salt and pepper: as needed
- Fresh parsley for garnish

How to Prepare: Olive oil should be heated in a big skillet to a temperature that is somewhere in the middle. A minute or so after including the smashed garlic, the garlic should become fragrant. After including the shrimp to the skillet, season them with smoky paprika, dried thyme, salt, and pepper. Sauté the shrimp for approximately 2 to 3 minutes on all sides, or until they become pink and opaque. Pour in lemon juice and stir in lemon zest. Cook for further minute to allow the flavors to meld. Put the shrimp on a platter that is intended for presenting. In the event that you so desire, garnish with freshly sliced parsley and additional lemon zest.

Nutritional Info: Calories: 190kcal, Protein: 24g, Carbohydrates: 2g, Dietary Fiber: 0g, Sugars: 1g, Fat: 9g, Saturated Fat: 1g, Cholesterol: 192mg, Sodium: 185m

7. Butternut Squash and Spinach Risotto

This is a creamy, satisfying dish perfect for a light lunch. The combination of roasted butternut squash and fresh spinach not only offers delightful flavor but also packs a nutritional punch. It's heart-healthy, supports digestion with its high fiber content, and is a great choice for maintaining a balanced diet while keeping calorie intake moderate.

(Ready in: 10 mins | Cook Duration: 30 mins | Persons: 4)

Necessary Items:

- 1/2 cup Arborio rice
- 2 cups low-sodium vegetable or chicken broth
- 3/4 cup butternut squash, skinned and cubed
- 1 cup fresh spinach leaves
- 1/2 small onion, finely cubed
- 1 piece garlic, crushed

- 2 tbsps dry white wine (elective)
- 1 tbsp olive oil
- 1/4 cup grated Parmesan cheese
- 1/8 tsp ground nutmeg
- Salt and pepper as needed
- Fresh sage leaves for garnish (elective)

How to Prepare: Warm up the oven to 400 deg.F (200 deg.C). The butternut squash cubes should be tossed with a 1/2 tbsp of olive oil, some salt, and some pepper beforehand. Put on a baking sheet and roast for 20 to 25 minutes, or until soft and slightly caramelized, whichever comes first. Keep the broth at a warm temperature by heating it in a saucepan at low temp. To warm the rest of the olive oil, put it in a big skillet or pan and set the middling temp. Approximately 2 minutes after including the cubed onion, the onion should become transparent. Cook for one more minute after stirring in the garlic that has been crushed. The Arborio rice should be added to the skillet and cooked for 2 minutes while being stirred continuously until the edges of the rice become transparent. When you are ready to use white wine, pour it in immediately and mix it until the majority of it has evaporated.

Make sure to start including the hot broth in the rice in increments of one ladle at a time. Be sure to stir the mixture often and wait for each addition to be absorbed prior to including the next. This should take about 18-20 minutes. When the rice is almost done, fold in the roasted butternut squash and fresh spinach. Cook until the spinach is wilted and the risotto is creamy. Stir in the grated Parmesan cheese and ground nutmeg. Salt and pepper should be used to adjust the seasoning. Garnish with fresh sage leaves if desired. Present instantly.

Nutritional Info: Calories: 310 kcal, Protein: 8g, Carbohydrates: 48g, Fat: 10g, Saturated Fat: 3g, Cholesterol: 10mg, Sodium: 650mg, Potassium: 550mg

---

8. Chickpea and Carrot Stew with Couscous

This stew is not only nutritious but also easy to digest and packed with flavors that can make a balanced diet enjoyable. The chickpeas provide a good source of plant-based protein and fiber, which are essential for maintaining muscle mass and promoting digestive health. Carrots contribute beta-carotene, supporting eye health and boosting immunity. The inclusion of almonds adds healthy fats and vitamin E, which can support heart health and cognitive function.

(Prep Time: 15 minutes | Cook Time: 30 minutes | Servings: 2)

Ingredients:

- 1 tbsp olive oil
- 1 medium onion, severed
- 2 pieces garlic, crushed
- 1 tsp ground cumin
- 1 tsp ground coriander
- 1/2 tsp ground cinnamon
- 1/2 tsp ground turmeric
- 1 cup canned cubed tomatoes
- 1 cup cooked chickpeas (canned or boiled)
- 2 cups vegetable broth
- 2 medium carrots, skinned and cubed
- 1/4 cup dried apricots, severed
- 1/4 cup almonds, cut
- 1 cup cooked couscous
- Fresh parsley for garnish

Instructions: Warm up the olive oil in a big saucepan by heating it at a middling temp. Include the severed onion and continue to sauté it until it becomes translucent and tender. Stir in the crushed garlic along with cumin, coriander, cinnamon, and turmeric, cooking until fragrant. Include cubed tomatoes, cooked chickpeas, vegetable broth, and cubed carrots. To prepare the carrots, bring the mixture to a simmer and continue cooking for around 15 minutes. Stir in the dried apricots that have been severed and continue to boil for a further 5 minutes. Present the stew over cooked couscous and garnish with sliced almonds and fresh parsley.

Nutritional Info: Calories: 370kcal | Protein: 12g | Fat: 7g | Saturated Fat: 1g | Cholesterol: 0mg | Sodium: 600mg | Carbohydrates: 64g | Fiber: 12g | Sugar: 23g

---

9. Chicken Salad with Walnuts and Grapes

This dish is a nutritious choice that supports both heart and overall health while being easy to prepare and enjoy. The chicken provides a lean source of protein, crucial for maintaining muscle mass and overall strength. Walnuts contribute heart-healthy fats and omega-3 fatty acids, which support cardiovascular health and cognitive function. Grapes include antioxidants, which can help combat inflammation and support cellular health. Additionally, the salad's combination of yogurt and mayonnaise provides a creamy texture without excessive calories.

(Ready in: 25 min | Cook Duration: 25 min | Persons: 2)

Necessary Items:

For the Filling:

- 2 tsps mayonnaise
- 1/3 Granny Smith apple, cut into small chunks
- 2 tsps creamy salad dressing
- 1/3 cup severed walnuts, or as needed
- 1/2 stalk celery, severed
- 1 1/2 tsps lemon juice
- 1 tbsp vanilla yogurt
- 2/3 cooked chicken breast, shredded
- 1/3 red onion, severed

3 seedless red grapes, divided

How to Prepare: The apple chunks, red onion, walnuts, shredded chicken, celery, and lemon juice should all be mixed together in a big mixing bowl at the same time. The vanilla yogurt, salad dressing, and mayonnaise should be combined in a small basin and mixed together. To ensure that the chicken mixture is properly coated, pour this mixture over it and stir it. Gently toss in the divided grapes. Present instantly or refrigerate until ready to eat.

Nutritional Info: Calories: 220kcal, Protein: 19g, Carbohydrates: 10g, Dietary Fiber: 2g, Sugars: 7g, Fat: 14g, Saturated Fat: 2g, Cholesterol: 55mg, Sodium: 130mg, Potassium: 300mg

10. Cauliflower Noodle Casserole

This casserole fits well into an intermittent fasting regimen, offering essential nutrients and satiety without excessive calories. Cauliflower provides a high-fiber, low-calorie base, supporting digestive health and weight management. Greek yogurt includes protein and probiotics, which are beneficial for muscle maintenance and gut health. The combination of cheese and olive oil ensures a satisfying meal that supports overall well-being while keeping calorie counts in check.

(Prep Time: 20 minutes | Cook Time: 35 minutes | Servings: 2)

Ingredients:

- 1 big head of cauliflower, cut into small florets and processed into "noodles"
- 1 tbsp olive oil
- Salt and black pepper, as needed
- 1/4 cup shredded cheddar cheese
- 3 oz. plain Greek yogurt
- 8 oz. tomato sauce
- Minced garlic, as needed
- A pinch of dried basil

Instructions: Prepare your oven to 400 deg.F (200 deg.C). Within a big skillet, bring the olive oil to a middling temp. Include the cauliflower noodles and cook until tender and slightly browned, around 5-7 minutes, including crushed garlic as desired. Repeat with any remaining cauliflower if needed. Prepare the mixture by combining tomato sauce, Greek yoghurt, dried basil, salt, and black pepper in a pot and heating it at low temp. Within 3 to 5 minutes, stir the sauce until it is entirely heated through.

After the cauliflower noodles have been cooked, put them in a baking dish. After pouring the tomato sauce mixture over the top, do a little toss to blend the components. A uniform layer of shredded cheddar cheese should be sprinkled over the top. In an oven that has been prepared, cook the cheese for 20 to 25 minutes, or until it is melted and bubbling.

Nutritional Info: Calories: 190kcal, Protein: 11g, Fat: 10g, Carbohydrates: 14g, Fiber: 5g, Sugar: 7g, Sodium: 290mg

11. Mediterranean Shrimp Salad with Lemon Tahini Dressing

For men over 60, this salad is an excellent choice. It's packed with protein from the shrimp, which supports muscle maintenance, while the fresh vegetables provide essential vitamins and fiber for digestive health. The healthy fats from the olive oil and tahini help improve heart health, making this dish a nutritious option, especially for those practicing intermittent fasting.

(Prep Time: 15 minutes | Cook Time: 5 minutes | Servings: 4)

Ingredients:

- 1 lb. big shrimp, skinned and deveined
- 2 cups mixed salad greens
- 1 cup cherry tomatoes, divided
- 1 cup cucumber, cubed
- 1/2 red onion, finely cut
- 1/4 cup Kalamata olives, pitted and cut
- 1/4 cup crumbled feta cheese
- Lemon wedges for presenting

For Lemon Tahini Dressing:

- 1/4 cup tahini
- 1/2 tsp ground cumin
- 2 tbsps lemon juice
- 1 tbsp honey
- 1 tbsp olive oil
- 1 tsp garlic powder
- Salt and pepper, as needed
- 2 tbsps water (adjust for desired consistency)

Instructions: Put the entire components for the lemon tahini dressing into a small bowl and whisk them together until they are entirely smooth. Depending on the situation, adjust the consistency with water. Include salt and pepper in the shrimp before cooking them. The shrimp should be fried in a pan at med-high temp. for approximately 2 to 3 minutes on all sides, or until they are pink and cooked all the way through. The mixed salad greens, cherry tomatoes, cucumber, red onion, and Kalamata olives should be combined together in a big bowl. Include the cooked shrimp to the salad. Include the lemon tahini dressing that has been prepared in the salad and toss it. Garnish the salad with crumbled feta cheese and lemon wedges. Present instantly and enjoy!

Nutritional Info: Calories: 330kcal | Protein: 27g | Fat: 18g | Saturated Fat: 3g | Cholesterol: 214mg | Sodium: 750mg | Carbohydrates: 14g | Fiber: 5g | Sugar: 6g

12. Zucchini Noodles with Spicy Peanut Sauce

Rich in healthy fats from peanut butter and sesame oil, this dish promotes heart health and provides long-lasting energy—ideal for those on an intermittent fasting regimen. The zucchini noodles keep it light and low in carbs while still providing essential fiber and nutrients.

(Ready in: 20 minutes | Cook Duration: 5 minutes | Persons: 2)

Necessary Items:

- Zucchinis, medium-sized: 2
- Peanut butter: 1/4 cup (creamy or chunky)
- Soy sauce: 2 tbsps (low-sodium recommended)
- Rice vinegar: 1 tbsp
- Sesame oil: 1 tsp
- Sriracha or chili paste: 1 tsp (adjust for spice level)
- Garlic piece: 1 (crushed)
- Lime juice: 1 tbsp
- Water: 2-3 tbsps (to thin sauce as needed)
- Salt and pepper: as needed
- Optional garnish: severed peanuts, cilantro, and lime wedges

How to Prepare: Spiralize the zucchinis into noodle-like strands using a spiralizer or julienne peeler. Set the zucchini noodles on paper towels to absorb extra moisture. In a medium bowl, whisk together peanut butter, soy sauce, rice vinegar, sesame oil, Sriracha (or chili paste), crushed garlic, and lime juice. The necessary consistency can be achieved by slowly including water, and then seasoning the mixture with salt and pepper. To get the sesame oil ready, heat a small amount of it in a big skillet at a temperature that is somewhere in the middle. The zucchini noodles should be added and cooked for 2 to 3 minutes until they have become somewhat softer but are still a little crispy. Take out from temp. and toss the zucchini noodles in the spicy peanut sauce until evenly coated. Present instantly, garnished with severed peanuts, fresh cilantro, and lime wedges for an extra burst of flavor.

Nutritional Info: Calories: 350 kcal, Protein: 10g, Carbohydrates: 15g, Dietary Fiber: 4g, Sugars: 6g, Fat: 28g, Saturated Fat: 5g, Cholesterol: 0mg, Sodium: 420mg, Potassium: 650mg

13. Spicy Sweet Potato and Black Bean Quinoa Bowl

This Spicy Sweet Potato and Black Bean Quinoa Bowl is perfect for men over 60, particularly those interested in maintaining heart health and stable energy levels. The combination of complex carbs from quinoa and sweet potatoes, along with the plant-based protein from black beans, ensures sustained energy throughout the day. The added spinach and bell pepper boost antioxidant intake, essential for overall vitality in later years.

(Ready in: 15 minutes | Cook Duration: 30 minutes| Persons: 2)

Necessary Items:

- Sweet potatoes, cubed: 2 cups
- Black beans (15 oz can), drained and washed: 1 can
- Quinoa, cooked: 2 cups
- Olive oil: 2 tbsps
- Chili powder: 1 tsp
- Ground cumin: 1/2 tsp
- Garlic powder: 1/2 tsp
- Salt and pepper: as needed
- Red bell pepper, cubed: 1 cup
- Fresh spinach: 2 cups, lightly wilted
- Optional topping: crumbled feta or queso fresco
- Optional garnish: fresh cilantro and lime wedges

How to Prepare: Warm up your oven to 400 deg.F (200 deg.C). To prepare the sweet potatoes, put them in a bowl and include the following components: olive oil, chili powder, cumin, garlic powder, salt, and pepper. After spreading them out equally on a baking sheet, roast them for 25 to 30 minutes, or until they are soft and mildly crunchy. A small amount of olive oil should be heated in a skillet, and the spinach should be wilted very slightly while the sweet potatoes are roasting. Set aside. Assemble your bowl by layering cooked quinoa at the base, followed by roasted sweet potatoes, black beans, and cubed red bell pepper. Top with the wilted spinach, crumbled feta or queso fresco, and fresh cilantro. Include a squeeze of lime juice for a zesty finish.

Nutritional Info: Calories: 450 kcal, Protein: 13g, Carbohydrates: 68g, Dietary Fiber: 14g, Sugars: 6g, Fat: 15g, Saturated Fat: 3g, Cholesterol: 5mg, Sodium: 360mg, Potassium: 900mg

14. Greek-Style Chicken Salad Bowl

Rich in lean protein from chicken and packed with Mediterranean superfoods like olives, feta, and greens, this dish promotes cardiovascular health while offering anti-inflammatory benefits. The yogurt-based tzatziki dressing adds probiotics, supporting digestive health—an essential aspect of healthy aging.

(Ready in: 15 minutes | Cook Duration: 15 minutes | Persons: 2)

Necessary Items:

- Grilled chicken breasts, finely cut: 2 pieces (alternatively, pre-cooked chicken or rotisserie chicken can be used)
- Olive oil: 1 tbsp
- Lemon juice: 1 tbsp
- Salt and pepper: as needed
- Mixed greens or arugula: 2 cups
- Cherry tomatoes, divided: 1 cup
- Cucumber, finely cut: 1 cup
- Kalamata olives, divided: 1/2 cup
- Crumbled feta cheese: 1/4 cup
- Red onion, finely severed: 1/4 cup
- Toasted pine nuts: 2 tbsps
- Fresh dill, severed: 2 tbsps

- For dressing: Greek yogurt-based tzatziki sauce (2 tbsps plain Greek yogurt, 1 tsp lemon juice, crushed garlic, dill, cucumber, salt, and pepper)

How to Prepare: If using pre-cooked chicken, slice it thinly. If grilling fresh chicken, flavor with salt, pepper, and lemon juice, then cook in olive oil at middling temp. until done (around 6-7 minutes on all sides). Let rest before slicing. Arrange the mixed greens or arugula as the base of your salad bowl. Include the divided cherry tomatoes, cut cucumber, Kalamata olives, crumbled feta, and finely severed red onion. Put the sliced chicken over the salad, making it the centerpiece of the dish. Drizzle with the homemade tzatziki dressing, giving the salad a creamy and tangy touch. Top with toasted pine nuts and fresh dill for an extra layer of flavor.

Nutritional Info: Calories: 410 kcal, Protein: 32g, Carbohydrates: 13g, Dietary Fiber: 4g, Sugars: 5g, Fat: 24g, Saturated Fat: 7g, Cholesterol: 105mg, Sodium: 470mg, Potassium: 620mg

15. Bell Peppers Stuffed with Quinoa, Spinach, and Feta

This dish offers a vibrant mix of flavors and nutrients. It is rich in fiber, antioxidants, and plant-based proteins, perfect for men over 60 seeking heart-healthy and anti-inflammatory meals. The combination of quinoa, spinach, and sun-dried tomatoes supports digestion and helps maintain muscle strength, making it an ideal choice for aging adults.

(Ready in: 15 minutes | Cook Duration: 40 minutes | Persons: 2)

Necessary Items:

- 2 big bell peppers (any color)
- 1/2 cup cooked quinoa
- 1/4 cup cooked spinach (drained)
- 1/4 cup crumbled feta cheese
- 2 tbsps severed sun-dried tomatoes
- 2 tbsps severed green onions
- 1 piece garlic, crushed
- 1/2 tbsp olive oil
- 1/2 tsp dried oregano
- Salt and pepper as needed
- Juice of 1/2 lemon
- Fresh parsley for garnish

How to Prepare: Warm up the oven to 375 deg.F (190 deg.C). Take out the seeds from the bell peppers and slice off the tops of the peppers. In a small baking dish, arrange them in an upright position. The quinoa that has been cooked, the spinach, the crumbled feta, the sun-dried tomatoes, the green onions, the smashed garlic, the olive oil, the oregano, the salt, and the pepper should be combined in a bowl before being included to the other components. Blend the lemon juice thoroughly after squeezing it in. Every bell pepper should be stuffed with the quinoa mixture. Put the dish in the oven for half an hour with the foil covering it. Take out the cover from the peppers and continue baking them for another 10 minutes, or until they reach the level of tenderness that you choose. You should present it warm and garnish it with fresh parsley.

Nutritional Info: Calories: 320 kcal, Protein: 11g, Carbohydrates: 42g, Fat: 13g, Fiber: 8g, Sodium: 520mg

16. Caper and Bean Salad with Tuna

This dish provides a great source of protein and fiber, which is critical for muscle health and digestion, especially for men over 60. The beans and tuna offer heart-healthy benefits, while the addition of fresh dill and radishes adds a burst of flavor and nutrients. This salad is both satisfying and beneficial, fitting well into a balanced diet.

(Ready in: 15 minutes | Persons: 2)

Necessary Items:

- 1 can of white beans (drained and washed, 15 oz)
- 1 can of tuna (drained, 5 oz)
- 1/2 cup cherry tomatoes, divided
- 1/4 cup cucumber, cubed
- 2 tbsps capers, washed
- 2 tbsps fresh dill, severed
- 1 tbsp red wine vinegar
- 1 tbsp extra-virgin olive oil
- 1/2 tsp dried thyme
- Salt and black pepper, as needed
- Optional: Sliced radishes, for garnish

How to Prepare: After combining the white beans, tuna, cherry tomatoes, cucumber, and capers in a big bowl, stir the components together. To form the dressing, take a small bowl and mix together the olive oil, red wine vinegar, dried thyme, salt, and pepper. Blend the components together until they are completely combined. Carefully toss the bean mixture after drizzling it with the dressing to ensure that it is uniformly coated. Garnish with fresh dill and, if desired, cut radishes for added crunch and color. Present instantly or chill for 15 minutes to allow the flavors to blend.

Nutritional Info: Calories: 290kcal, Protein: 22g, Carbohydrates: 28g, Dietary Fiber: 9g, Sugars: 3g, Fat: 12g, Saturated Fat: 2g, Cholesterol: 30mg, Sodium: 680mg, Potassium: 650mg

17. Roasted Cauliflower and Broccoli Gratin

This Roasted Cauliflower and Broccoli Gratin brings a comforting twist to classic vegetables. The rich blend of Gruyère and Parmesan cheeses adds a flavorful, creamy touch, while the Greek yogurt and mayonnaise enhance the texture and boost the protein content. The inclusion of roasted vegetables provides essential vitamins and minerals, beneficial for maintaining bone health and overall vitality. High in fiber and low in sugars, this gratin supports digestive health and is a great option for men over 60 who are aiming to balance flavor with nutritional benefits.

(Ready in: 20 minutes | Cook Duration: 30 minutes | Persons: 2)

Necessary Items:

- 1/2 head cauliflower, cut into florets
- 1/2 head broccoli, cut into florets
- 1 tbsp olive oil
- 1 small shallot, finely cubed
- 1 piece garlic, crushed
- 1/2 cup shredded Gruyère cheese

- 1/4 cup grated Parmesan cheese
- 1/4 cup Greek yogurt
- 1/4 cup mayonnaise
- 1/2 tsp Dijon mustard
- 1/4 tsp dried rosemary
- Salt and black pepper, as needed
- 2 tbsps panko breadcrumbs
- Severed chives, for garnish

How to Prepare: Warm up the oven to 375 deg.F (190 deg.C). Grease a small baking dish with a light coating. Olive oil, salt, and pepper should be mixed with the cauliflower and broccoli florets before being tossed. They should be roasted for 15 minutes, or until they begin to turn brown, after being spread out on a baking pan. The shallot and garlic should be cooked in a skillet with a little bit of olive oil until they become fragrant and tender. In a bowl, mix the shredded Gruyère cheese, grated Parmesan, Greek yogurt, mayonnaise, Dijon mustard, dried rosemary, and cooked shallot and garlic. Use pepper and salt to season the food. The roasted vegetables should be combined with the cheese mixture and then stirred until they are completely coated. Transfer to the baking dish that has been prepared. Panko breadcrumbs should be sprinkled on top, and the dish should be baked for 20 minutes, or until the top is brown and crispy. Garnish with severed chives before serving.

Nutritional Info: Calories: 390 kcal, Protein: 15g, Carbohydrates: 20g, Dietary Fiber: 6g, Sugars: 7g, Fat: 27g, Saturated Fat: 12g, Cholesterol: 55mg, Sodium: 540mg, Potassium: 750mg

18. Spinach and Goat Cheese Omelette

This Spinach and Goat Cheese Omelette is a delicious, protein-rich dish that's perfect for a quick and satisfying meal. For men over 60, it provides high-quality protein to support muscle maintenance and bone health, while the spinach offers a boost of vitamins and minerals. The inclusion of goat cheese adds a creamy texture and a unique flavor, along with a bit of calcium.

(Ready in: 15 minutes | Cook Duration: 15 minutes | Persons: 2)

Necessary Items:

- 1 tbsp olive oil
- 1/2 small onion, finely cubed
- 4 big eggs
- 1/4 cup milk
- Salt and black pepper, as needed
- 2 oz. goat cheese, crumbled
- 1 cup fresh spinach, severed
- 1 tbsp fresh chives, severed (for garnish)

How to Prepare: In a skillet that does not stick, bring the olive oil to a middling temp. In around 3 to 4 minutes, include the cubed onion and continue to sauté it until it becomes translucent and tender. Cook for a further 1 to 2 minutes after including the severed spinach until it has wilted. Eggs and milk should be mixed together in a bowl using a whisk. Use pepper and salt to flavor the food. Pour the egg mixture into the skillet, stirring gently to blend with the onions and spinach. Sprinkle crumbled goat cheese evenly over the top.

The omelette should be allowed to cook without being disturbed for around 3 to 4 minutes, or until the sides have become firm but the center is still mildly runny. Carefully fold the omelette in half and cook for further 1-2 minutes, or until fully set. Garnish with fresh chives before serving.

Nutritional Info: Calories: 280 kcal, Protein: 16g, Carbohydrates: 5g, Dietary Fiber: 2g, Sugars: 3g, Fat: 22g, Saturated Fat: 8g, Cholesterol: 320mg, Sodium: 400mg, Potassium: 350mg

19. Avocado and Kale Soup

This soup is ideal for those who enjoy a creamy, satisfying dish without the need for cooking, and its chilled nature makes it especially refreshing. It's packed with healthy fats from avocado and olive oil, which are great for cardiovascular health—a key concern for men over 60. Kale adds a boost of vitamins A, C, and K, while Greek yogurt provides protein and probiotics for digestive health. The combination of fresh parsley and lemon juice not only brightens the flavor but also offers additional antioxidants.

(Ready in: 15 minutes | Persons: 2)

Necessary Items:

- 1 ripe avocado, skinned and pitted
- 1 cup kale, stems taken out and leaves severed
- 1/2 cup plain Greek yogurt
- 2 tbsps fresh parsley, severed
- 1 piece garlic, crushed
- 2 tbsps severed green onions
- 1/2 small cucumber, skinned and cubed
- 1 tbsp lemon juice
- 1 tbsp extra-virgin olive oil
- Salt and black pepper, as needed
- Optional garnish: Extra severed parsley, cubed cucumber, and a drizzle of olive oil

How to Prepare: Peel and pit the avocado. Rinse and chop the kale. In a mixer or food processor, blend the avocado, kale, Greek yogurt, parsley, crushed garlic, green onions, and cubed cucumber. Include the lemon juice and blend until smooth and creamy. While the blender is operating, gradually include the extra-virgin olive oil using a drizzling method until it is completely incorporated. Include some salt and black pepper according to preference and flavor with salt. To bring out the full range of flavors, the soup should be chilled in the fridge for almost 2 hours. Present chilled, garnished with additional parsley, cubed cucumber, and a splash of olive oil if desired.

Nutritional Info: Calories: 295kcal, Protein: 6g, Carbohydrates: 18g, Dietary Fiber: 8g, Sugars: 4g, Fat: 24g, Saturated Fat: 4g, Cholesterol: 2mg, Sodium: 70mg, Potassium: 880mg

20. Tropical Mango and Chicken Lettuce Wraps

For men over 60, this dish offers several benefits. The lean chicken and high fiber from the vegetables and mango support heart health and aid in digestion. The low-calorie nature of lettuce wraps helps with weight management, while the vitamins in mango and vegetables contribute to overall cognitive function and eye health.

(Ready in: 20 minutes | Cook Duration: 10 minutes | Persons: 2)

Necessary Items:

For the Lettuce Wraps:

- 1 cup cooked chicken breast, shredded or cubed
- 1 ripe mango, skinned and cubed
- 1/2 cup shredded carrots
- 1/2 small red bell pepper, finely cut
- 1/4 cup finely severed red onion
- 1 tbsp fresh cilantro, severed
- 4 big lettuce leaves (e.g., iceberg or butter lettuce)

For the Tropical Dressing:

- 1 tbsp lime juice, freshly squeezed
- 1 tbsp extra-virgin olive oil
- 1 tsp honey
- 1 tsp soy sauce
- 1/2 tsp ground cumin
- Salt and black pepper, as needed

How to Prepare: If using pre-cooked chicken, shred or dice it into bite-sized pieces. If cooking fresh chicken, flavor with salt and pepper and cook in a skillet at middling temp. with a small amount of olive oil until fully cooked. After it has cooled, the chicken should be shredded or diced. Diced mango, shredded carrots, sliced red bell pepper, severed red onion, and fresh cilantro should all be mixed together in a bowl before being added to the components. To ensure that the lime juice, olive oil, honey, soy sauce, ground cumin, salt, and pepper are thoroughly mixed together, put them in a small bowl and whisk them together. The shredded chicken should be combined with the tropical dressing in a big bowl at this point. Put the lettuce leaves on serving plates or a big platter. Spoon the chicken mixture and the mango-vegetable mixture onto the lettuce leaves. Garnish with additional cilantro if desired and present instantly as refreshing lettuce wraps.

Nutritional Info: Calories: 290 kcal, Protein: 22g, Carbohydrates: 27g, Dietary Fiber: 4g, Sugars: 14g, Fat: 12g, Saturated Fat: 2g, Cholesterol: 60mg, Sodium: 290mg

Chapter 7: Dinner Recipes For Intermittent Fasting

1. Honey Sesame Salmon

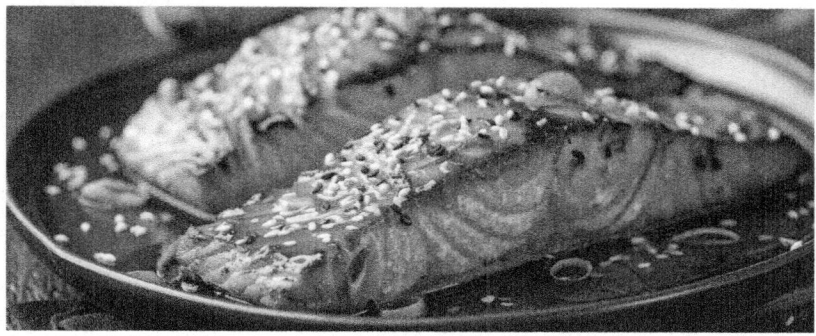

For those practicing intermittent fasting, this meal provides a satisfying source of protein and healthy fats that can help maintain muscle mass and keep you feeling full longer. The balance of protein and carbs also supports stable energy levels post-fast, making it an ideal choice to break your fast while promoting overall health. Salmon, which is abundant in omega-3 fatty acids, is a good food for maintaining a healthy heart.

(Prep Time: 20mins | Cook Time: 20mins | Serves: 2)

Ingredients:

- Pepper: for sprinkling
- Salt: for sprinkling
- Salmon fillets: 1 lb.
- Honey: 1/4 cup
- Water: 1/4 cup

- Sesame oil: 2 tbsps
- Soy sauce: 2 tbsps
- Garlic, crushed: 2 pieces
- Lemon juice: juice of 1 lemon
- Cornstarch: 1/2 tsp, dissolved in a small amount of water

Instructions: Warm up the oven to 375 deg.F (190 deg.C). Flavor the salmon with salt and pepper, then bake it for 20 minutes (cook time may vary depending on fillet size). Meanwhile, blend water, lemon juice, honey, sesame oil, soy sauce, and crushed garlic in a saucepan. The mixture should be brought to a boil. Allow the sauce to continue cooking until the corn flour mixture has thickened it. Present the sauce with the baked salmon.

Nutritional Info: Calories: 470kcal, Protein: 31.7g, Carbohydrates: 34g, Fat: 13.2g, Saturated Fat: 2.5 g, Cholesterol: 89 mg, Sodium: 446.7 mg, Sugars: 30 g, Potassium: 832 mg

2. Honey Garlic Tofu

This Honey Garlic Tofu is a tasty and heart-healthy dish, offering plant-based protein ideal for men over 60. It's packed with antioxidants and low in saturated fats, helping to support cardiovascular health. In a regimen of intermittent fasting, this dish provides essential nutrients and balanced energy to keep you feeling satisfied post-fast, promoting muscle maintenance and overall vitality.

(Ready in: 15mins | Cook Duration: 5mins | Persons: 2)

Necessary Items:

- Firm tofu: 1/2 lb. (about 225 g), pressed and cubed
- Soy sauce: 2 tbsps
- Olive oil: 1.5 tsps
- Green onion: severed, for garnish
- Honey: 2 tbsps + 2 tsps
- Garlic pieces: 1, crushed
- Minced ginger: 1/2 tsp

How to Prepare: In a medium mixing bowl, blend the honey, soy sauce, garlic, and ginger. Half of this mixture will be used for the marinade, and the other half will be used to cook the tofu. Put the tofu cubes in a big sealable container or bag. Pour half of the marinade/sauce mixture on top, gently mix, and let the tofu marinate for 15 minutes or up to 8 hours in the fridge. Cover and refrigerate the remaining marinade. At medium-high temp., bring the olive oil to a simmer in a saucepan. Throw away the marinade that was used and include the tofu that has been marinated in the skillet. To achieve a golden and crispy texture, cook for a couple of minutes on all sides. Once the rest of the marinade or sauce has been poured in, continue to boil the tofu for another couple of minutes, until it is coated and caramelized. Present with brown rice and steamed veggies, garnished with green onion.

Nutrition: Cal: 270, Total Fat: 8g, Carb: 25g, Dietary Fiber: 3g, Sugars: 23g, Protein: 20g, Sodium: 520mg, Potassium: 190 mg

---

3. Pork Tenderloin Stuffed with Apple, Walnuts, and Sage

Pork tenderloin is a lean protein that helps maintain muscle mass, which is crucial as we age. The walnuts include healthy fats that support heart health, and the apples provide fiber and natural sweetness without including refined sugars. Sage offers anti-inflammatory benefits. This balanced meal supports both muscle recovery and sustained energy.

(Ready in: 25 minutes | Cook Duration: 35mins | Serving 2)

Necessary Items:

- Pork tenderloin (about 1 lb.): 1
- Apple, skinned and finely cubed: 1 medium
- Walnuts, severed: 1/4 cup
- Fresh sage, severed: 1 tbsp
- Garlic, crushed: 2 pieces
- Olive oil: 2 tbsps
- Salt and black pepper, as needed
- Cooking twine

How to Prepare: Warm up your oven to 375 deg.F (190 deg.C). The olive oil, which is 1 tbsp, should be heated in a skillet at a middling temp. Include the garlic and sauté it for around a minute, or until it becomes fragrant. To the skillet, include the apple that has been diced, the walnuts that have been severed, and the fresh sage. Cook for 3 to 4 minutes, or until the apples have made a small softening and the mixture has been thoroughly blended. Use pepper and salt to flavor the food. To create a butterfly pattern on the pork tenderloin, slice it lengthwise, taking care not to cut it all the way through into the center. It should be opened up and then flattened with a meat mallet. Both salt and pepper should be used to season the interior of the pork. The pork should be rolled up firmly and secured with cooking twine once the apple and walnut mixture has been spread evenly over the pig slices. In a skillet that can go in the oven, raise the temperature of the rest of the olive oil to medium-high settings. For approximately 3 minutes on all sides, sear the pork until it is browned on both sides. Bake the pan for 20 to 25 minutes, or until the internal temp. reaches 145 deg.F (63 deg.C), once the oven has been warmed. Prior to slicing the pork, allow it to rest for 5 to 10 minutes. Present and take pleasure in it!

Nutritional Info: Cal: 380, Total Fat: 20g, Carb: 12g, Fiber: 3g, Sugars: 8g, Protein: 35g

4. Roasted Carrots with Garlic and Herb Infusion

Simple yet satisfying, this recipe helps maintain balanced nutrition and supports overall well-being. The carrots provide a rich source of beta-carotene, vital for eye health, while the olive oil adds heart-healthy fats. The garlic and herbs bring a flavorful punch without including unnecessary calories, making it a nutrient-dense choice for breaking a fast.

(Ready in: 10 mins | Cook Duration: 20 mins | Persons: 2)

Necessary Items:

- Carrots, skinned and cut into sticks or rounds: 2 cups
- Olive oil: 2 tbsps
- Fresh thyme or rosemary, severed: 1 tbsp
- Garlic, crushed: 2 pieces
- Salt and black pepper, as needed
- Lemon juice: 1 tbsp
- Severed fresh parsley (elective, for garnish)

How to Prepare: Set your oven to 400 deg.F (200 deg.C). Carrots, olive oil, garlic that has been smashed, and either fresh thyme or rosemary should be mixed together in a big mixing bowl. Include salt and black pepper as needed, then drizzle in the lemon juice for a zesty twist. Toss the carrots until they are well coated. Arrange the carrots in a single layer on a baking sheet that has been covered with parchment paper. Bake them for 15 to 20 minutes, tossing them regularly, until they are cooked and have a tiny crunch to them. Take out of the oven and place on a tray specifically designed for presenting. Adding freshly cut parsley as a garnish will include a splash of color and flavor to the dish.

Nutritional Info: Cal: 160, Fat: 10g, Carb: 14g, Dietary Fiber: 4g, Sugars: 6g, Protein: 2g

5. Herb-Crusted Baked Haddock

This recipe is light on carbs and full of essential nutrients, making it a smart choice for a balanced meal after fasting. The lean protein from the haddock supports muscle health, while the yogurt and Parmesan mixture provides rich flavor without excess calories.

(Ready in: 35mins | Serves: 2)

Ingredients:

- 1/2 cup grated Parmesan cheese
- 2 tbsps freshly squeezed lemon juice
- 2 tbsps Greek yogurt
- 2 tbsps severed fresh parsley
- 1.5 tbsps crushed garlic

- 2 tbsps unsalted butter, softened
- 1/4 tsp dried thyme
- 1/8 tsp lemon zest
- 1/4 tsp paprika
- A dash of Dijon mustard

Instructions: Warm up your oven to 350 deg.F (175 deg.C). Lightly grease an 8x8-inch baking dish with butter. Lay the haddock fillets in a single layer in the dish, ensuring they're not overlapping. Drizzle the fillets with lemon juice, ensuring the tops are evenly coated. In a small bowl, blend Parmesan cheese, softened butter, Greek yogurt, crushed garlic, parsley, thyme, paprika, lemon zest, and a dash of Dijon mustard. Mix thoroughly until you have a smooth, creamy mixture. Once the haddock fillets have reached the point where they can be easily flaked apart with a fork, bake them for 10 to 20 minutes, based on the thickness of the fillets. Once the baking dish has been removed from the oven, spread the cheese mixture over the fillets in a uniform consistency. Please put the dish back into the oven and continue baking for a further 5 minutes, or until the topping is bubbling and brown in color. Present with roasted vegetables, quinoa, or a fresh salad for a light and nutritious meal.

Nutritional Info: Calories: 330kcal, Protein: 32g, Carbohydrates: 5g, Fat: 20g, Saturated Fat: 9g, Cholesterol: 115mg, Sodium: 540mg, Fiber: 0.5g, Sugar: 1g

6. Citrus-Basil Baked Cod with Roasted Cherry Tomatoes

Rich in protein and low in carbohydrates, this dish supports muscle maintenance and overall health while keeping energy levels steady. The combination of cod and tomatoes offers beneficial omega-3 fatty acids and antioxidants, which are particularly advantageous for men over 60. These nutrients support heart health and cognitive function, making it an ideal choice for a balanced, fasting-friendly diet.

(Ready in: 10mins | Cook Duration: 20mins Persons: 2)

Necessary Items:

- 2 cod fillets (6-8 oz each)
- 1 pint cherry tomatoes
- 3 garlic pieces, crushed
- 1 tbsp fresh basil, severed
- 1 tbsp fresh thyme, severed

- 2 tbsps avocado oil
- Salt and black pepper, as needed
- 1 tbsp lemon zest
- Lemon wedges for garnish

How to Prepare: Warm up your oven to 400 deg.F (200 deg.C). A mixture of cherry tomatoes, crushed garlic, fresh basil, fresh thyme, and avocado oil should be mixed together in a mixing dish. Flavor with salt and black pepper, and then toss the components together until they are well distributed. Once the cod fillets have been seasoned with salt and pepper, place them on a baking tray that has been prepped with parchment paper. Bake for around 30 minutes. The lemon zest should be sprinkled over the fillets. The tomato mixture should be spread around the cod fillets that are placed on the baking pan. The cod should be cooked for 15 to 20 minutes, or until it is soft and readily flakes apart with a fork, and the tomatoes should be roasted and overflowing with flavor. Lemon wedges should be used as a garnish prior to presenting. You may present this dish with a side of steamed veggies or a quinoa salad that is on the lighter side.

Nutritional Info: Calories: 310, Fat: 14g, Carb: 9g, Dietary Fiber: 2g, Sugars: 5g, Protein: 36g

---

7. Grilled Lemon Garlic Chicken Breasts

This recipe not only provides lean protein essential for muscle maintenance and repair but also incorporates fresh lemon and garlic, known for their health benefits. Lemon is high in vitamin C, which supports immune health and improves collagen production, while garlic has been shown to have anti-inflammatory properties and may help with heart health. For men on intermittent fasting, this meal supports sustained energy levels and provides essential nutrients without excess calories.

(Ready in: 30 minutes - including marinating time - | Cook Duration: 10 mins | Persons: 2)

Necessary Items:

- 2 boneless, skinless chicken breasts
- 2 tbsps olive oil
- Juice and zest of 1 lemon
- 3 garlic pieces, crushed
- 2 tbsps fresh rosemary, severed
- 1 tsp dried thyme
- Salt and black pepper, as needed
- Lemon wedges for garnish

How to Prepare: Take the chicken breasts and begin by preparing them. To make a tasty marinade, include the following ingredients in a mixing bowl: olive oil, lemon juice, lemon zest, crushed garlic, severed rosemary, dried thyme, salt, and pepper. The chicken breasts should be placed in a plastic bag that can be sealed or a shallow dish, and then half of the marinade should be poured over them. Put the mixture in the fridge for almost 15 minutes with the lid or cover it so that the flavors can blend. First, bring your grill or grill pan up to a temp. of medium-high. The chicken should be removed from the marinade, and any excess should be allowed to drain off before placing it on the grill. Grill the chicken for approximately five minutes on all sides, or until it reaches an internal temp. of 165 deg.F (74 deg.C) and is attractively blackened. Please allow the chicken to rest for a couple of minutes after it has been cooked prior to cutting it. Present the grilled chicken breasts with lemon wedges for an extra zing. This dish pairs wonderfully with a side of steamed vegetables or a light salad.

Nutritional Info: Calories: 320, Fat: 18g, Carbs: 5g, Dietary Fiber: 1g, Sugars: 2g, Protein: 36g

8. Maple-Balsamic Glazed Chicken Thighs with Roasted Butternut Squash

This meal provides a rich source of protein from the chicken thighs, which helps maintain muscle mass and support metabolic health. The butternut squash adds essential vitamins and fiber, promoting digestive health and sustained energy. The combination of maple syrup and balsamic vinegar offers a flavorful yet balanced approach to reducing added sugars, making this dish ideal for those focusing on a low-carb, nutrient-dense diet during their eating window.

(Ready in: 30 mins – plus marinating time - | Cook Duration: 25 mins | Persons: 2)

Necessary Items:

For the Chicken Thighs:

- 4 bone-in, skinless chicken thighs (about 1 lb or 450g)
- 1/4 cup balsamic vinegar
- 1/4 cup pure maple syrup
- 2 tbsps Dijon mustard
- 2 pieces garlic, crushed
- 1 tsp dried rosemary
- Salt and black pepper, as needed
- 2 tbsps olive oil

For the Roasted Butternut Squash:

- 2 cups butternut squash, skinned and cubed
- 1 tbsp olive oil
- 1/2 tsp dried thyme
- Salt and black pepper, as needed

How to Prepare: FOR THE CHICKEN THIGHS: Whisk together the following ingredients in a small bowl: balsamic vinegar, maple syrup, Dijon mustard, crushed garlic, dried rosemary, and a pinch of salt and black pepper. The chicken thighs should be placed in a plastic bag that can be sealed or a shallow dish, and then half of the marinade should be spilled over them. To achieve a more robust flavor, marinate the chicken in the fridge for almost half an hour, but preferably for up to 2 hours. Warm up your oven to 400 deg.F (200 deg.C). At medium-high temp., warm the olive oil in a big skillet that can be used in the oven. Around 4 to 5 minutes, sear the chicken thighs with the skin-side down until they are golden brown. After turning the chicken over, douse it with the remaining marinade and set it aside. After placing the skillet in the oven, roast the chicken for 20 minutes, or until the internal temp. of the chicken reaches 165 deg.F (74 deg.C). FOR THE ROASTED BUTTERNUT SQUASH: The butternut squash cubes should be tossed with olive oil, dried thyme, salt, and black pepper while the chicken is coming to a roasting temperature. Put the squash on a baking sheet in a single layer and set it over the oven. Bake for approximately 20 to 25 minutes, or until the meat is tender and has a light caramelization. To present, plate the chicken thighs alongside the roasted butternut squash. Drizzle any pan juices over the chicken for extra flavor. Enjoy this hearty and flavorful meal, perfect for a balanced diet.

Nutritional Info: Calories: 400, Fat: 18g, Carb: 30g, Fiber: 5g, Sugars: 15g, Protein: 30g

9. Citrus-Dijon Salmon with Roasted Cauliflower and Carrots

This meal provides a great balance of protein from the salmon, which supports muscle health and overall vitality, while the citrus-Dijon glaze adds flavor with minimal sugars. The roasted cauliflower and carrots contribute essential vitamins and fiber, aiding digestion and keeping you full longer. This dish fits well into a low-carb, nutrient-rich eating window, helping maintain energy and health.

(Ready in: 15 min – plus marinating time - | Cook Duration: 25 min | Persons: 2)

Necessary Items:

For the Citrus-Dijon Salmon:

- Salmon fillets (approximately 6 oz/170g each): 2
- Fresh orange juice: 2 tbsps
- Dijon mustard: 1 tbsp
- Honey: 1/2 tbsp
- Minced garlic pieces: 1
- Fresh dill, severed: 1/2 tbsp
- Salt and black pepper, as needed
- Olive oil: 1 tbsp

For the Roasted Cauliflower and Carrots:

- Cauliflower florets: 1 cup
- Carrots, skinned and sliced: 1/2 cup
- Olive oil: 1 tbsp
- Salt and black pepper, as needed
- Ground cumin: 1/2 tsp
- Fresh parsley, severed (elective): 1 tbsp

How to Prepare: FOR THE CITRUS-DIJON SALMON: A mixture of orange juice, honey, Dijon mustard, smashed garlic, fresh dill, salt, and black pepper should be mixed together in a basin using a whisk. A dish should be used to place the salmon fillets, and then half of the citrus-Dijon marinade should be poured over them. The rest of the marinade should be saved for later. For roughly 15 minutes, the salmon should be allowed to marinade. Preheat your oven to 375 deg.F (190 deg.C). In a skillet that can go in the oven, bring the olive oil to a medium-high temp. After adding the salmon fillets that have been marinated, place them with the skin side down (if they have skin) and sear them for 2 to 3 minutes till they create a golden crust. Salmon should be roasted for 12 to 15 minutes, or until it can be readily flaked apart with a fork, once the skillet has been transferred to the oven that has been warmed. FOR THE ROASTED CAULIFLOWER AND CARROTS: Olive oil, salt, black pepper, and ground cumin should be mixed together in a baking dish before being added to the cauliflower florets and carrot slices. Roast in the oven for approximately 20 to 25 minutes, tossing everything halfway through, until it is soft and caramelized. To prepare the dish for serving, arrange the roasted cauliflower and carrots on separate dishes. Top with a salmon fillet and drizzle with the reserved citrus-Dijon marinade. Garnish with fresh parsley if desired.

Nutritional Info: Calories: 430, Fat: 22g, Carb: 28g, Fiber: 7g, Sugars: 14g, Protein: 35g

10. Herbed Chicken with Swiss Cheese

The combination of chicken and Swiss cheese provides a high amount of lean protein, which supports muscle maintenance and overall strength. The addition of thyme and turkey bacon offers a burst of flavor with minimal added sodium. This dish is low in carbohydrates and high in protein, making it a perfect fit for a low-carb, nutrient-dense eating window.

(Prep Time: 5mins | Cook Time: 25 mins | Servings: 2)

Ingredients:

- 2 slices Swiss cheese
- 1/8 tsp paprika
- 2 thin slices turkey bacon or low-sodium ham
- Olive oil spray

- 4 fresh thyme sprigs
- 2 boneless skinless chicken breast halves (about 4 oz. each)
- Salt and black pepper, as needed

Instructions: Salt, black pepper, and paprika should be used to flavor the chicken breasts at this point. Prepare a big skillet by spraying it with olive oil spray and heating it over medium-high temp. Cook the chicken breasts in the skillet for approximately 4 to 5 minutes on all sides, or until the internal temp. reaches 165 deg.F. Transfer the cooked chicken breasts to an ungreased baking sheet. Top each chicken breast with 2 fresh thyme sprigs and 1 slice of turkey bacon (or low-sodium ham). The chicken breasts should each have one slice of Swiss cheese placed on top of them. Cook the chicken breasts under the broiler for a couple of minutes, or until the cheese is melted and bubbling, at a distance of 6 to 8 inches from the heat source.

Nutritional Info: Calories: 290kcal | Carbohydrates: 2g | Protein: 43g | Fat: 13g | Sodium: 530mg | Fiber: 0g | Sugar: 1g

11. Ricotta and Sun-Dried Tomato Stuffed Salmon

This recipe blends the richness of salmon with the creamy filling of ricotta, spinach, and sun-dried tomatoes, creating a balanced meal that's packed with healthy fats, lean protein, and vibrant flavors. For men over 60 who are practicing intermittent fasting, this dish is ideal because it provides a satisfying, nutrient-dense meal that promotes muscle maintenance, supports heart health with omega-3 fatty acids, and includes fiber to aid digestion. The combination of protein and healthy fats also helps maintain satiety, which is crucial for managing hunger during fasting periods.

(Ready in: 20 minutes | Cook Duration: 25 minutes | Persons: 2)

For the Stuffed Salmon:

- 2 salmon fillets (about 6 oz/170g each)
- 1/2 cup ricotta cheese
- 1/4 cup sun-dried tomatoes, severed
- 1/4 cup spinach, severed

- 2 tbsps grated Parmesan cheese
- 1 garlic piece, crushed
- 1/2 tsp dried thyme
- Salt and black pepper, as needed

For the Lemon Herb Butter Sauce:

- 2 tbsps butter
- 1 garlic piece, crushed
- Juice of 1/2 lemon
- Zest of 1/2 lemon
- 1 tbsp severed fresh parsley
- Salt and black pepper, as needed

How to Prepare: For the Stuffed Salmon: Warm up your oven to 375 deg.F (190 deg.C). Ricotta cheese, sun-dried tomatoes, spinach, Parmesan cheese, crushed garlic, dried thyme, salt, and pepper should be mixed together in a basin. Blend thoroughly. Each salmon fillet should have a pocket created by cutting a horizontal slit down the side of the fillet. Stuff each fillet with the ricotta and sun-dried tomato mixture, pressing gently to close the pocket. Flavor the outside of the salmon with salt and pepper. Apply a small amount of olive oil to a skillet that does not stick and heat it over medium-high temp. About 2 to 3 minutes on all sides, sear the salmon fillets that have been packed until they are golden brown. When the salmon is done being seared, transfer it to a baking dish and bake it in an oven that has been warmed for 15 to 20 minutes, or until it can be easily flaked with a fork. **For the Lemon Herb Butter Sauce:** Melt the butter in the same skillet that was used to sear the salmon over a cooking of middling temp. Continue to sauté the garlic mince for a couple of minutes until it becomes aromatic. Once the mixture has been removed from the heat, toss in the lemon juice, lemon zest, and Severed parsley. Use pepper and salt to flavor the food. **To present:** Spoon the lemon herb butter sauce over the stuffed salmon fillets and present instantly, accompanied by your favorite side dishes.

Nutritional Info: Calories: 420, Total Fat: 26g, Carb: 6g, Fiber: 2g, Sugars: 3g, Protein: 38g

12. Coconut Curried Pumpkin Soup

This dish is packed with anti-inflammatory ingredients such as turmeric and ginger, which are beneficial for men over 60. The healthy fats from coconut milk and the fiber-rich pumpkin make this a nourishing, filling meal ideal for intermittent fasting. This soup supports digestion, offers antioxidants, and provides sustained energy, all while being light on calories to help with weight management and overall health.

(Ready in: 10 minutes | Cook Duration: 30 minutes | Persons: 2)

Necessary Items:

- 2 cups pumpkin, skinned and cubed (or canned pumpkin puree)
- 1 small onion, severed
- 1 tbsp olive oil
- 1/2 tsp curry powder
- 1/4 tsp ground cinnamon
- 1/4 tsp ground turmeric
- 1/4 tsp ground cumin
- 2 pieces garlic, crushed
- 1 tbsp crushed fresh ginger
- 2 cups vegetable broth
- 1/2 cup coconut milk
- Salt and black pepper, as needed
- Fresh cilantro or pumpkin seeds, for garnish (elective)

How to Prepare: Olive oil should be heated in a medium-sized pot at a middling temp. Chop the onion and sauté it for 2 to 3 minutes, or until it becomes translucent. Continue to simmer for an additional couple of minutes after including the ginger and garlic that has been crushed. Curry powder, ground cinnamon, ground turmeric, and ground cumin should be stirred in at this point. Toast the spices for about 1 minute to release their flavors. Include the cubed pumpkin to the pot, tossing it with the spice mixture for 2-3 minutes until well coated. After that, pour in the coconut milk and the vegetable broth. Turn the heat down to a low setting when the mixture has been brought to a boil. For 20 to 25 minutes, or until the pumpkin is soft, cover and boil the mixture. The soup should be blended with care using either an immersion blender or a conventional blender until it is completely smooth and creamy. Make sure to season it to taste with salt and black pepper, and then continue to simmer for another 5 minutes. Use a ladle to transfer the coconut curry pumpkin soup into dishes. In the event that you so prefer, garnish with fresh cilantro or pumpkin seeds. Warm the dish.

Nutritional Info: Calories: 210, Fat: 13g, Carb: 22g, Dietary Fiber: 6g, Sugars: 7g, Protein: 3g

13. Eggplant Parmesan with Spinach and Avocado Salad

This Eggplant Parmesan is a lighter, plant-based take on the classic dish, perfect for men over 60. Eggplant provides antioxidants and fiber, while the healthy fats from avocado and olive oil support heart health and satiety—crucial for maintaining energy levels during intermittent fasting. This meal offers a satisfying balance of protein, fiber, and essential nutrients to keep you nourished while supporting weight management and metabolic health.

(Prep Time: 20 minutes | Cook Time: 40 minutes | Servings: 2)

Ingredients:

For the Eggplant Parmesan:

- 1 medium eggplant, cut into 1/2-inch rounds
- 1 cup marinara sauce
- 1/2 cup panko breadcrumbs
- 1/4 cup grated Parmesan cheese
- 1 egg, beaten
- 1/2 tbsp olive oil

For the Spinach and Avocado Salad:

- 2 cups fresh spinach leaves
- 1/2 avocado, cubed
- 1/2 tbsp lemon juice
- 1/2 tbsp extra-virgin olive oil
- Salt and black pepper, as needed

Instructions: For the Eggplant Parmesan: Warm up the oven to 375 deg.F (190 deg.C). After coating all slices of eggplant with panko breadcrumbs that have been combined with grated Parmesan cheese, the eggplant slices are dipped in the beaten egg. Arrange the eggplant slices that have been coated on a baking sheet that has been covered with parchment paper. Sprinkle a little bit of olive oil on top. Sauté the eggplant slices in the oven for 20 to 25 minutes, or until they are soft and golden brown. At the same time, bring the marinara sauce to a simmer at middling temp. until it is completely warmed. **For the Spinach and Avocado Salad:** To prepare the salad, blend the cubed avocado and spinach in a big bowl. Include the lemon juice, extra-virgin olive oil, salt, and black pepper to the salad. **To Present:** Plate the baked eggplant Parmesan with the warm marinara sauce on the side. Present alongside the fresh spinach and avocado salad.

Info: Calories: 320kcal, Carb: 28g, Protein: 13g, Fat: 17g, Sodium: 640mg, Fiber: 8g, Sugars: 6g

14. Lemon Rosemary Grilled Swordfish

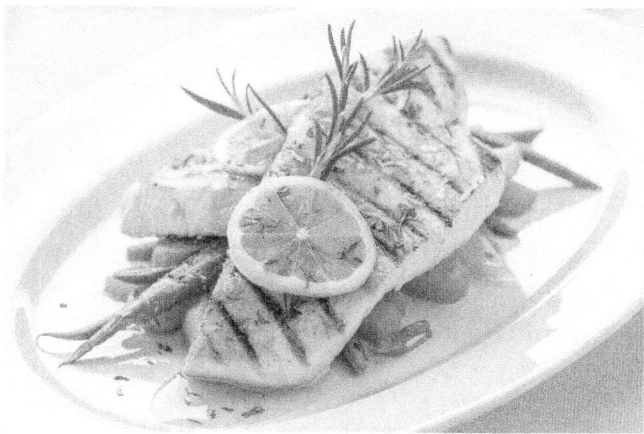

This dish is a flavorful and nutritious option, perfect for men over 60 practicing intermittent fasting. Swordfish is rich in lean protein and omega-3 fatty acids, which support heart health and muscle maintenance. The light, zesty marinade of lemon and rosemary adds a burst of antioxidants, while the low-carb profile helps maintain steady energy levels without spiking insulin.

(Ready in: 15 minutes, Cook Duration: 10-12 minutes, Persons: 4)

Necessary Items:

- Swordfish fillets (4, about 6 oz. each)
- Zest and juice of 1 lemon
- Minced garlic (2 pieces)
- Finely severed fresh rosemary (2 tbsps)
- Olive oil (2 tbsps)
- Salt and black pepper, as needed
- Lemon wedges
- Fresh rosemary sprigs (elective)

How to Prepare: In your most cherished petite bowl, craft a zesty symphony using bright lemon zest, tangy lemon juice, aromatic crushed garlic, fresh-cut rosemary, a drizzle of olive oil, and a dash each of salt and black pepper. This magical potion is the secret song for your swordfish! Lay your majestic swordfish fillets in a graceful dance arena, be it a dish or a zip-top bag. Pour the freshly crafted citrus song over them, ensuring every inch bathes in its melodies. Cloak the dish or seal the song within the bag and send it to the chill chambers (refrigerator) for a brief 15-minute ballad of flavors. Fire up your grill, aiming for a passionate medium-high embrace (around 400 deg.F or 200 deg.C). Gently brush the grill grates with love and oil to ensure a smooth dance floor for the fish. Bid farewell to the marinade and gently dab the swordfish with paper towels, preparing them for their spotlight moment. Let the swordfish groove on the grill for a captivating 5-6 minutes on all sides. Their readiness is marked by easy flaking and charming grill tattoos. Remember, their dance might be shorter or longer depending on their thickness. With grace, escort the perfectly grilled swordfish to their final resting stage, a beautiful serving platter. Adorn with lemony crescents and rosemary wands for an encore presentation. Present while the applause (heat) is still high, and let the taste buds revel in the celebration!

Nutritional Info: Calories: 290, Fat: 12g, Carb: 3g, Fiber: 1g, Sugars: 0g, Protein: 42g

15. Grilled Lamb Chops with Basil Pesto and Roasted Sweet Potatoes

This meal strikes a balance between rich flavors and essential nutrients, promoting vitality and wellness for those embracing a healthy fasting routine. Lamb provides high-quality protein essential for muscle preservation, while basil and parsley offer antioxidant benefits. Sweet potatoes include complex carbohydrates for sustained energy and fiber, supporting digestive health during fasting windows.

(Prep Time: 15 minutes, Cook Time: 25 minutes, Servings: 2)

Ingredients:

For the Lamb Chops:

- 2 boneless lamb chops (about 6 oz each)
- 1 tbsp olive oil
- Salt and pepper as needed

For the Roasted Sweet Potatoes:

- 1 medium sweet potato, skinned and cubed
- 1/2 tbsp olive oil
- Salt and pepper as needed

For the Basil Pesto:

- 1/4 cup fresh basil leaves, severed
- 1/4 cup fresh parsley, severed
- 1 piece garlic, crushed
- 2 tbsps walnuts, toasted

- 1/4 cup extra-virgin olive oil
- 1 tbsp lemon juice
- Salt and pepper as needed

Instructions: Prepare the Basil Pesto: The severed basil, parsley, garlic that has been crushed, and walnuts that have been toasted should be combined in a food processor. Pulse until extremely finely crushed. While it is operating, gradually include the olive oil and lemon juice until the mixture is completely smooth. Include salt and pepper as needed, and flavor with salt. Put away for later. **Flavor and Grill the Lamb Chops:** First, bring the grill up to a medium-high temp. Apply olive oil, salt, and pepper to the lamb chops, and then rub them in. Grill for 3 to 4 minutes on all sides, or until the meat reaches the desired level of doneness. Take away and allow to relax. **Roast the Sweet Potatoes:** Warm up the oven to 425 deg.F (220 deg.C).

Olive oil, salt, and pepper should be mixed with the sweet potatoes that have been Severed. A baking sheet should be used to lay them out in a single layer. To achieve a soft and golden brown texture, roast for 20 minutes. **Present:** Plate the grilled lamb chops with a generous spoonful of basil pesto on top. Present alongside the roasted sweet potatoes.

Info: Calories: 370kcal, Carb: 22g, Protein: 26g, Fat: 20g, Sodium: 230mg, Fiber: 4g, Sugars: 5g

16. Sweet Potato and Rosemary Risotto

This dish offers a comforting and hearty meal that's perfect for IF. Sweet potatoes provide complex carbohydrates and fiber, which help sustain energy levels throughout your eating window. Rosemary adds a fragrant touch and may offer cognitive benefits, which is particularly valuable for men over 60. This dish also delivers a good amount of protein and essential vitamins, supporting overall health while adhering to a balanced intermittent fasting regimen.

(Ready in: 10 minutes | Cook Duration: 30 minutes | Persons: 2)

Necessary Items:
- 3/4 cup Arborio rice
- 2 cups chicken or vegetable broth
- 1/2 cup pureed sweet potato
- 1/4 cup dry white wine (elective)
- 1/2 small onion, finely severed
- 1 piece garlic, crushed
- 1 tbsp olive oil
- 1 tbsp fresh rosemary, severed
- 1/4 cup grated Pecorino cheese
- Salt and black pepper, as needed
- Fresh rosemary sprigs for garnish

How to Prepare: While the broth is being heated in a pot at low temp., it should be kept warm. Prepare the olive oil by heating it in a big skillet at a middling temp. The onion should be cooked for 2 to 3 minutes until it becomes transparent. Garlic that has been crushed and Arborio rice should be added to the skillet and cooked for 2 to 3 minutes, or until the rice has a light toasty flavor. If you are using white wine, pour it in and mix it until it is almost completely absorbed. Starting with a ladleful at a time, pour the warm broth to the rice while turning it often before including more. Before proceeding to the following addition, be sure that each one has been digested. Cook for approximately 20 minutes, or until the rice is creamy and has a firm texture. Blend in the pureed sweet potato and the rosemary that has been cut. Continue to cook for another 2 to 3 minutes until everything is thoroughly mixed and cooked through. After taking the dish off the heat, toss in the shredded Pecorino cheese. Include some salt and black pepper as needed and season with salt. Present in bowls, garnished with fresh rosemary sprigs.

Nutritional Info: Cal: 350, Fat: 11g, Carbohydrates: 55g, Fiber: 7g, Sugars: 8g, Protein: 10g

17. Herbed Spaghetti Squash with Roasted Bell Peppers and Feta

With its low-calorie profile and high fiber content, this dish helps keep you full longer while providing essential nutrients. The combination of roasted bell peppers and feta adds flavor and protein, supporting muscle health and overall wellness, making it a great choice for men over 60. Enjoy this nourishing meal as part of a balanced intermittent fasting regimen.

(Ready in: 15 minutes | Cook Duration: 40 minutes | Persons: 2)

Necessary Items:

- 1 small to medium spaghetti squash
- 1/2 cup roasted red bell peppers, severed (store-bought or homemade)
- 1/4 cup crumbled feta cheese
- 1 tbsp olive oil
- 1/2 tbsp fresh oregano leaves, severed
- 1/2 tbsp fresh basil leaves, severed
- Salt and black pepper, as needed
- Fresh basil leaves for garnish

How to Prepare: Warm up your oven to 375 deg.F (190 deg.C). A longitudinal cut should be made in the spaghetti squash, and the seeds should be removed. Olive oil should be used to coat the sliced sides of the squash, and then salt and black pepper should be applied to the squash. Arrange the squash halves on a baking sheet that has been covered with parchment paper, with the cut side facing down. The squash should be roasted in the oven for 30 to 40 minutes, or until it is tender and can be readily shredded using a food processor. It is recommended that you prepare the roasted bell peppers while the squash is roasting. Chop them into bite-sized pieces if using store-bought. If roasting your own, roast and peel them before chopping. When the squash is done cooking, take it out of the oven and allow it to cool down for a short while. Make the flesh into strands that resemble spaghetti by shredding it with a fork. It is recommended to heat a small amount of olive oil in a big skillet at middling temp. Put in the roasted bell peppers and continue to cook them for 2 to 3 minutes, or until they are completely hot. Include the shredded spaghetti squash to the skillet, tossing to blend with the peppers. Stir in the fresh oregano and basil, allowing them to wilt slightly.

Take out from temp. and sprinkle with crumbled feta cheese. Flavor with additional salt and pepper if needed. Present in bowls, garnished with fresh basil leaves for a burst of flavor.

Nutritional Info: Calories: 270, Fat: 19, Carbohydrates: 23g, Fiber: 5g, Sugars: 7g, Protein: 7g

18. Walnut-Crusted Turkey Cutlets

The combination of crunchy walnut coating and tender turkey provides a satisfying, nutrient-rich meal. High in protein and healthy fats, this dish supports muscle maintenance and heart health, which are particularly beneficial for men over 60. As a result of its low carbohydrate content, which helps to maintain stable blood sugar levels, this is an excellent option for maintaining your sense of fullness and energy levels throughout your fasting period.

(Ready in: 15 minutes | Cook Duration: 15 minutes | Persons: 4)

Necessary Items:

- Turkey cutlets (4, about 1 lb.)
- Finely severed walnuts (1 cup)
- Whole wheat breadcrumbs (1/2 cup)
- Grated Parmesan cheese (1/4 cup)
- Severed fresh parsley (2 tbsps)
- Dried thyme (1 tsp)
- Eggs (2)
- Olive oil (2 tbsps)
- Salt and black pepper, as needed

For Serving (elective):

- Lemon wedges

How to Prepare: In a dish that's just the right depth, summon walnuts, breadcrumbs, the majestic Parmesan, vibrant parsley, and the ever-so-aromatic dried thyme. Include a touch of salt and pepper for a little extra zing, then blend them into a harmonious mix. In a neighboring dish, create a pool of whipped dreams by beating the eggs into submission. Flavor those turkey cutlets! A sprinkle of salt and pepper does wonders for their personality. Take each turkey artist and dip them into our egg whirlpool, ensuring they are glistening from edge to edge. Without hesitation, introduce them to the nutty ensemble, ensuring they wear their walnut wardrobe with pride. Set the stage with olive oil in a skillet at medium-high fire. Await its beckoning call - that shimmer that says, "It's showtime." With grace, lay each walnut-adorned turkey cutlet on the stage. Let them dance for about 3-4 minutes on all sides, aiming for a finale of golden brown perfection. Once their performance ends, escort the turkey stars onto a paper towel carpet to bask, ensuring they retain only the good kind of oils. Present these Walnut Wonders steaming and, for an added flourish, let lemon wedges grace their side.

Nutritional Info: Calories: 380, Fat: 24g, Carb: 10g, Fiber: 2g, Sugars: 1g, Protein: 33g

19. Ginger-Lime Chicken with Cucumber and Bell Pepper Salad

This meal is both flavorful and balanced, aiding in sustained energy levels and overall well-being during your eating period. The lean chicken provides high-quality protein to support muscle health, while the bell pepper adds a boost of vitamin C and antioxidants.

(Prep Time: 15 minutes | Cook Time: 15 minutes | Servings: 2)

Ingredients:

- 2 chicken breasts (about 6 oz each)
- 2 tbsps lime juice
- 1 tbsp low-sodium soy sauce
- 1 tbsp honey
- 1 tbsp freshly grated ginger
- 1 piece garlic, crushed
- 1 tbsp olive oil
- 1/2 cucumber, finely cut
- 1/2 red bell pepper, finely cut
- 1/4 cup severed fresh cilantro
- Salt and black pepper, as needed

Instructions: To make a marinade, blend lime juice, honey, soy sauce, grated ginger, and crushed garlic in a small bowl. Mix well. The chicken breasts should be placed in a shallow dish, and then half of the marinade should be poured over them. Marinate for almost 10 minutes, turning occasionally. At medium-high temp., bring the olive oil to a simmer in a pan. To ensure that the chicken breasts are completely done, grill them for 6-7 minutes on all sides after marinating them. While the chicken cooks, blend cucumber slices, bell pepper slices, and severed cilantro in a bowl. Toss with the remaining marinade, and season with salt and pepper. Slice the cooked chicken and present it alongside the cucumber and bell pepper salad.

Nutritional Info: Calories: 330kcal, Carb: 15g, Protein: 35g, Fat: 17g, Sodium: 350mg

20. Stuffed Zucchini with Quinoa and Turkey

This dish provides lean protein from turkey and quinoa, supporting muscle maintenance and sustained energy. The zucchini serves as a low-carb, nutrient-rich base, while goat cheese adds a creamy touch with reduced fat content. High in fiber and essential vitamins, this meal supports digestive health and helps keep you full during fasting periods.

(Ready in: 30 minutes, Cook Duration: 45mins, Persons: 2)

Necessary Items:

- 4 medium zucchinis
- 2 boneless, skinless turkey breasts, cubed
- 1/2 cup cooked quinoa
- 1/4 cup crumbled goat cheese
- 1/4 cup severed sun-dried tomatoes (packed in oil)
- 1/4 cup severed fresh basil
- 1/4 cup severed red onion
- 1 piece garlic, crushed
- 1 tbsp olive oil
- 1 tsp dried basil
- Salt and pepper, as needed
- 1/2 cup chicken broth
- Lemon wedges, for presenting (elective)

How to Prepare: Set to 375 deg.F (190 deg.F). In order to make boats, cut the zucchinis in half lengthwise and take out the seeds from the center of all sides. They should be placed in a baking dish. Prepare the olive oil by heating it in a skillet at medium-high temp. The turkey should be roasted until it is browned and cooked through, which should take around 5 to 6 minutes. Salt, pepper, and dried basil should be used as seasonings. Stir in cooked quinoa, crumbled goat cheese, severed sun-dried tomatoes, fresh basil, severed red onion, and crushed garlic. Mix well. Spoon the turkey and quinoa mixture into the zucchini boats, packing it tightly. Pour chicken broth into the bottom of the baking dish. After covering the zucchinis with foil, bake them for 30 to 35 minutes, or until they are soft. On the occasion that you so wish, garnish with more fresh basil and lemon wedges. Warm the dish.

Nutritional Info: Calories: 425, Fat: 15g, Carb: 40g, Fiber: 6g, Sugars: 5g, Protein: 35g

Chapter 8: Snack & Dessert Recipes For Intermittent Fasting

1. Coconut Chia Pudding with Mango

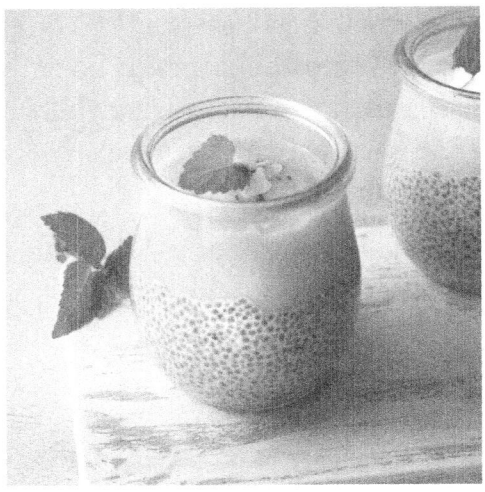

Combining the creamy texture of coconut milk with the fiber-packed chia seeds and the sweetness of ripe mango, this dish offers numerous benefits for men over 60. The chia seeds provide essential omega-3 fatty acids and fiber, promoting heart health and aiding in digestion. Coconut milk adds a dose of healthy fats, while mango contributes vitamins A and C, supporting immune function and skin health.

(Ready in: 10mins | Persons: 2)

Necessary Items:

- Chia seeds: 1/4 cup
- Coconut milk: 1 cup
- Honey or maple syrup (elective, for sweetness): 1 tbsp
- Vanilla extract: 1/2 tsp
- Ripe mango, cubed: 1
- Fresh mint leaves for garnish (elective)

How to Prepare: Dive into a bowl and conjure up a tropical potion by mingling chia seeds, the embrace of coconut milk, nature's sweet drizzle (honey or maple syrup), and a whisper of vanilla. Stir this magic until the chia seeds dance in unison. Let this concoction dream for a mere 5 minutes, but disturb its slumber after the first minute for a quick swirl, ensuring no chia seed feels left out. Cloak the bowl and let it slumber in the icy chambers of your fridge. Let the dreams last for 2 hours or a night-long voyage. In this time, the chia seeds will sip on the elixir and morph into a pudding sorcery. As the grand serving moment approaches, court a ripe mango into surrendering its golden cubes. Gently awaken your chilled chia creation, giving it a hearty stir. If it's too lost in its dreams, a splash more of coconut milk will bring it back to reality. Pour the chia enchantment into regal glasses or bowls, ready for the feast. Crown each serving with the golden mango treasures. For an added touch of magic, let fresh mint leaves sprinkle their blessings. Revel in this chilled tropical delight!

Nutritional Info: Calories: 235 kcal, Carbohydrates: 24g, Fiber: 9g, Sugars: 10g, Protein: 5g, Fat: 15g, Saturated Fat: 11g, Cholesterol: 0mg, Sodium: 14mg

---

2. Peanut Butter Oatmeal Chocolate Chip Cookies

Packed with healthy fats and protein, these cookies support muscle maintenance and heart health, crucial for men over 60. The fiber from oats aids digestion and helps regulate blood sugar levels, making these cookies a beneficial choice for those following an intermittent fasting regimen.

(Ready in: 15 minutes | Cook Time: 25min | Persons: 15)

Necessary Items:

- 1 cup rolled oats
- 1/2 cup creamy peanut butter
- 1/2 cup dark chocolate chips
- 1/4 cup honey or maple syrup
- 1 egg
- 1/2 tsp baking soda
- 1/4 cup severed walnuts (elective)
- 1/2 tsp vanilla extract

How to Prepare: Warm up the oven to 175 deg.C (350 deg.F). Place parchment paper on a baking pan and set it aside. Whisk the egg and peanut butter together in a big bowl until the mixture is completely smooth. The honey or maple syrup, baking soda, and vanilla extract should be stirred in at this point. Include the chocolate chips and rolled oats, and if you want to include walnuts, mix them in until they are well incorporated. Disperse tablespoons of dough onto the baking sheet that has been prepared, leaving about an inch of space between each one. Applying the back of the spoon, slightly flatten each of the patties. Bake the cookies for 12 to 15 minutes, or until the centers are firm and the edges have a color that is somewhere between golden brown and brown. It is recommended that the cake be allowed to cool for 10 minutes on the baking sheet before being moved to a wire rack to complete the cooling process.

Nutritional Info: Calories: 140kcal, Carbohydrates: 15g, Fiber: 2g, Sugars: 8g, Protein: 5g, Fat: 7g, Saturated Fat: 1g, Cholesterol: 10mg, Sodium: 100mg

---

3. Spiced Almond-Coconut Energy Bites

The spices not only enhance flavor but also contribute to anti-inflammatory benefits. Almonds provide protein and healthy fats, supporting muscle health and cardiovascular function. Shredded coconut adds fiber and a touch of natural sweetness, while dates offer a quick energy boost.

(Ready in: 20mins | Serves: 12)

Ingredients:

- 1 cup almonds
- 1 cup shredded unsweetened coconut
- 1/2 cup dates, pitted
- 2 tbsps almond butter
- 1 tbsp honey (or maple syrup for a vegan option)
- 1/2 tsp ground cinnamon

- 1/4 tsp ground nutmeg
- Pinch of sea salt

Instructions: In a food processor, blend almonds and shredded coconut. Pulse until finely ground. Include dates, almond butter, honey, cinnamon, nutmeg, and a pinch of sea salt to the processor. Blend until the mixture sticks together when pressed. Roll the mixture into 12 small balls, about 1 inch in diameter. Put the energy bites on a plate or tray covered with parchment paper. Refrigerate for 10 minutes to firm up before serving.

Nutritional Info: Cal: 130kcal, Protein: 4g, Carb: 10g, Fat: 15g, Fiber: 8g, Sugars: 8g

4. Avocado-Cocoa Mousse with a Hint of Mint

This dessert is naturally sweetened with maple syrup or honey, making it a lower-sugar option for intermittent fasting. Avocados provide healthy fats that support heart health and cognitive function, while cocoa adds a touch of antioxidants.

(Prep Time: 10 minutes | Chill Time: 2 hours | Servings: 4)

Ingredients:

- 2 ripe avocados
- 1/4 cup unsweetened cocoa powder
- 1/4 cup maple syrup or honey (adjust as needed)
- 1 tsp vanilla extract
- 2 tbsps almond milk (or any milk of choice)
- 1/4 tsp sea salt
- Fresh mint leaves for garnish (elective)

Instructions: Prepare a food processor by placing the flesh of the avocados inside of it. Put in some cocoa powder, some honey or maple syrup, some vanilla extract, some almond milk, and some salt from the sea. While blending, pause occasionally to scrape down the sides of the bowl to ensure that the mixture is fully smooth and creamy. In the event that it is required, adjust the sweetness as appropriate. To allow the mousse to solidify, put it in serving dishes and put them in the fridge for almost 2 hours. Garnish with fresh mint leaves before serving if desired.

Info: Cals: 210kcal | Fat: 15g | Protein: 3g | Sodium: 81mg | Carb: 19g | Fiber: 7g | Sugars: 9g

5. Baked Pears with Cinnamon and Pecans

Pears are rich in dietary fiber, aiding digestion and supporting heart health, while pecans provide healthy fats and antioxidants. This dessert fits well into intermittent fasting, offering a natural sweetness from honey and a dose of essential nutrients without overloading on sugars. Pairing with Greek yogurt or ricotta adds protein and a creamy texture, making it a balanced treat that supports overall wellness and fits within a healthy eating plan.

(Ready in: 15 minutes | Cook Duration: 25 minutes | Persons: 2)

Necessary Items:

- 2 ripe pears
- 2 tbsps honey
- 1/4 cup severed pecans
- 1/2 tsp ground cinnamon

- A pinch of nutmeg (elective)
- Greek yogurt or a dollop of ricotta cheese for presenting (elective)

How to Prepare: Warm up your oven to 350 deg.F (175 deg.C). Wash and halve the pears, removing the core and seeds with a spoon. In a small bowl, mix together honey, severed pecans, ground cinnamon, and a pinch of nutmeg if using. Put the pear halves cut-side up on a baking sheet or in a baking dish. Spoon the honey-pecan mixture into the hollow of each pear half. Bake in the warmed up oven for around 20-25 minutes, or until the pears are tender and caramelized. Allow the pears to cool slightly before serving. For an extra touch, top with a spoonful of Greek yogurt or ricotta cheese.

Nutritional Info: Calories: 220kcal, Carbohydrates: 33g, Protein: 3g, Fat: 10g, Saturated Fat: 1g, Cholesterol: 5mg, Sodium: 1mg, Fiber: 6g, Sugars: 23g

6. Carrot Oatmeal Raisin Muffins

For men over 60 practicing intermittent fasting, these muffins offer a balanced mix of protein, fiber, and healthy fats that support sustained energy levels and overall well-being. Carrots and oats provide essential vitamins and fiber, promoting digestive health and heart function. The Greek yogurt and oats also contribute to muscle maintenance and satisfaction during eating windows.

(Ready in: 15 minutes | Cook Duration: 20-25 minutes | Persons: 12)

Necessary Items:

- 1 cup all-purpose flour
- 1/2 cup whole wheat flour
- 1/2 cup granulated sugar
- 1/2 cup packed brown sugar
- 1 tsp baking powder
- 1/2 tsp baking soda
- 1/2 tsp salt
- 1 tsp ground cinnamon
- 1/4 tsp ground ginger
- 2 big eggs
- 1/2 cup unsalted butter, melted and cooled
- 1/4 cup plain Greek yogurt
- 1 tsp vanilla extract
- 1 cup grated carrot (about 2 medium carrots)
- 1/2 cup rolled oats
- 1/2 cup raisins

How to Prepare: Warm up your oven to 175 deg.C (350 deg.F). Paper liners should be used to line a muffin tin, or the cups should be lightly greased. Blend all-purpose flour, whole wheat flour, granulated sugar, brown sugar, baking powder, baking soda, salt, cinnamon, and ginger in a big mixing bowl. All of these components should be mixed together. To ensure a smooth mixture, stir. A separate bowl should be used to blend the eggs, melted butter, Greek yoghurt, and vanilla extract by whisking them together. To the dry mixture, include the liquid components and whisk until they are almost completely incorporated. Carrots that have been grated, rolled oats, and raisins should be folded in until they are spread equally.

The mixture should be distributed evenly among the muffin cups, and then each cup should be filled roughly two-thirds of the way at the top. The baked item should be baked for 20 to 25 minutes in an oven that has been warmed up, or until a toothpick that is put into the center of the baked good comes out clean or with only a few moist crumbs showing. When the muffins have reached the desired temperature, they should be allowed to cool for 5 minutes in the pan before being moved to a wire rack to complete the cooling process.

Nutritional Info: Calories: 230 kcal, Carbohydrates: 34g, Protein: 5g, Fat: 9g, Saturated Fat: 5g, Cholesterol: 35mg, Sodium: 200mg, Fiber: 3g, Sugars: 20g

7. Herbed Almonds with Rosemary

For men over 60 following intermittent fasting, these almonds provide a nutrient-dense, low-carb snack that can help maintain energy levels and support overall wellness. Almonds are packed with healthy fats, protein, and fiber, making them an excellent choice for satisfying hunger and supporting heart health. The addition of rosemary not only enhances flavor but also adds antioxidants.

(Ready in: 5 minutes | Freeze Time: 15 minutes | Persons: 4)

Necessary Items:

- 2 cups whole almonds
- 2 tbsps fresh rosemary leaves, severed
- 2 tbsps olive oil
- 1 tsp sea salt
- 1/2 tsp black pepper
- 1/4 tsp garlic powder (elective for extra flavor)

How to Prepare: Cover a baking sheet with parchment paper and warm up your oven to 325 deg.F (163 deg.C). Blend whole almonds with fresh rosemary, olive oil, sea salt, black pepper, and garlic powder, if using. Blend the entire ingredients together in a large mixing basin. Turn the almonds over until they are equally coated. The almonds should be spread out in a single layer on the baking sheet that has been prepared. Roast in an oven that has been warmed up for 15 minutes, tossing the mixture once or twice while it is cooking to ensure that it toasts evenly. Keep a cautious eye out to avoid getting burned. Take the bread out of the oven when it has reached a golden brown color and a pleasant aroma, and then wait for it to cool down before taking it from the baking sheet. As they cool, the almonds will acquire a more satisfying crunch. After the almonds have cooled, put them in a container that is sealed or present them right away.

Nutritional Info: Calories: 310kcal, Carbohydrates: 7g, Protein: 8g, Fat: 28g, Saturated Fat: 2.5g, Cholesterol: 0mg, Sodium: 580mg, Fiber: 4g, Sugars: 1g

8. Chocolate Avocado Pudding

For men over 60, this pudding provides heart-healthy fats from avocados, antioxidants from cocoa, and a good dose of fiber, which aids in digestion and helps manage blood sugar levels.

(Persons: 4 | Ready in: 10 minutes)

Necessary Items:

- Ripe avocados, skinned and pitted: 2
- Unsweetened cocoa powder: 1/4 cup
- Honey or maple syrup (adjust as needed): 1/4 cup
- Milk (dairy or non-dairy): 1/4 cup
- Vanilla extract: 1 tsp
- A pinch of salt
- Optional toppings: sliced strawberries, raspberries, severed nuts, or whipped cream

How to Prepare. The ripe avocados, unsweetened cocoa powder, honey or maple syrup, milk, vanilla extract, and a bit of salt should be mixed together in a food processor or blender. Puree the entire components until they are silky smooth and creamy. There is a possibility that you will need to scrape down the sides of the blender or food processor and blend once more in order to guarantee that there are no bits of avocado. After tasting the pudding, assess the level of sweetness and, if necessary, correct it by including additional honey or maple syrup. Once the mixture is smooth and sweetened to your liking, divide it into four serving cups or bowls. Refrigerate the Chocolate Avocado Pudding for almost 30 minutes to chill and firm up. Before serving, you can include your choice of toppings such as sliced strawberries, raspberries, severed nuts, or a dollop of whipped cream.

Nutritional Info: Calories: 237 kcal, Carbohydrates: 27g, Protein: 3g, Fat: 16g, Saturated Fat: 3g, Cholesterol: 0mg, Sodium: 37mg, Fiber: 7g, Sugars: 17g

9. Berry Chia Seed Smoothie

Combining a mix of blueberries, strawberries, and raspberries with the creamy texture of Greek yogurt and the nutrient-dense chia seeds, this smoothie packs a punch of antioxidants, fiber, and protein. For men over 60, this smoothie offers heart-healthy benefits from the berries, aids digestion with chia seeds, and supports muscle health with Greek yogurt.

(Persons: 2 | Ready in: 5 minutes)

Necessary Items:

- 1 cup mixed berries (blueberries, strawberries, raspberries)
- 1 ripe banana
- 2 tbsps chia seeds
- 1 cup Greek yogurt (or dairy-free yogurt for a vegan option)
- 1 cup unsweetened almond milk (or any preferred milk)
- Honey or agave syrup (elective, for sweetness)
- Ice cubes (elective)
- Fresh berries and mint leaves for garnish (elective)

How to Prepare: Blend the berries, banana, chia seeds, Greek yogurt, and almond milk in a blender. Include ice cubes if desired for a thicker, frostier texture. Blend until smooth. Adjust sweetness with honey or agave syrup if needed. Pour into glasses and garnish with extra berries and mint leaves if desired.

Nutritional Info: Calories: 250 kcal, Carbohydrates: 48g, Protein: 8g, Fat: 7g, Saturated Fat: 2g, Cholesterol: 6mg, Sodium: 70mg, Fiber: 9g, Sugars: 28g

10. Almond Butter Cookies

Made with almond butter, these cookies provide a good source of protein and healthy fats, making them an ideal snack for men over 60. The inclusion of almond butter supports heart health and offers a nutrient boost, while the cookies' balanced energy content fits well into an intermittent fasting regimen.

(Prep Time: 15 minutes | Cook Time: 10 minutes | Servings: 24)

Ingredients:

- 1 cup unsalted butter
- 1 cup almond butter
- 1 cup white sugar
- 1 cup packed brown sugar
- 2 big eggs
- 2 1/2 cups all-purpose flour
- 1 tsp baking powder
- 1 1/2 tsps baking soda
- 1/2 tsp salt

Instructions: The butter, almond butter, and both sugars should be creamed together in a mixing dish until the mixture is smooth and they are thoroughly blended. After including the eggs, continue to mix until they are thoroughly blended. A second bowl should be used to blend the flour, baking powder, baking soda, and salt by whisking them together. While continuing to mix, gradually incorporate the dry components into the liquid mixture until a dough is formed. The dough should be chilled for one hour in order to harden. Using parchment paper, line baking pans and warm up the oven to 375 deg.F (190 deg.C). Put the dough balls, which should be about one inch in diameter, on the baking pans that have been prepared. Make a crisscross pattern on each cookie by using a fork to create the pattern. The cookies should be baked for around 10 minutes, or until they have a golden brown color. The cookies should be allowed to cool for a couple of minutes on the baking pans before being transferred to a wire rack to finish cooling entirely.

Nutritional Info: Calories: 210kcal | Fat: 12g | Protein: 4g | Sodium: 190mg

11. Creamy Coconut Rice Pudding with Chia Seeds

This dish is a deliciously rich and wholesome dessert, made with coconut milk and chia seeds for an extra boost of healthy fats and fiber. It's a comforting, yet nutrient-dense option for men over 60, especially those practicing intermittent fasting. The coconut milk provides medium-chain triglycerides (MCTs), which support energy levels, while chia seeds include fiber and omega-3s to promote heart health and digestion.

(Persons: 4 | Ready in: 10 minutes | Cook Duration: 30 minutes)

Necessary Items:

- Arborio rice (or short-grain rice): 1 cup
- Coconut milk (full-fat or light): 4 cups
- Maple syrup or honey: 1/2 cup
- Chia seeds: 2 tbsps
- Vanilla extract: 1 tsp
- Pinch of salt

- Toasted coconut flakes and chia seeds for garnish (elective)

How to Prepare: Put the Arborio rice and 2 cups of coconut milk into a saucepan of medium size and continue cooking. For the purpose of preventing the mixture from sticking, bring to a simmer at middling temp. and whisk it constantly. Immediately after the mixture starts to simmer, turn the heat down to a low setting and continue cooking. The remaining coconut milk should be added carefully, perhaps half a cup at a time, while mixing often. After 15-20 minutes of cooking, stir in the maple syrup (or honey), chia seeds, vanilla extract, and a pinch of salt. Continue cooking, mixing regularly, until the rice is soft and the pudding has thickened, usually around 25-30 minutes total. Once done, take out from temp. and let the pudding rest for a couple of minutes. If the consistency is too dense, include a splash of coconut milk to loosen it up. Present warm or chilled, garnished with toasted coconut flakes and a sprinkle of chia seeds.

Nutritional Info: Calories: 360 kcal, Carbohydrates: 68g, Protein: 6g, Fat: 11g, Saturated Fat: 7g, Sodium: 95mg, Fiber: 4g, Sugars: 27g

12. Coconut Carrot Crunch Cookies

Perfect for men over 60, especially those on intermittent fasting, these cookies provide a boost of fiber and nutrients in a balanced, low-glycemic treat. The carrots offer a good source of vitamin A, promoting eye health, while coconut brings in healthy fats that support metabolism, making them an ideal snack between fasting windows.

(Persons: 24 cookies| Ready in: 15 minutes | Cook Duration: 15mins)

Necessary Items:

- 1 1/2 cups rolled oats
- 3/4 cup shredded coconut (unsweetened)
- 1 cup almond flour
- 1/2 tsp baking soda
- 1/2 tsp ground ginger
- 1/4 tsp salt
- 1/2 cup coconut oil, melted
- 1/4 cup maple syrup
- 1 big egg
- 1 tsp vanilla extract
- 1 cup grated carrot
- 1/4 cup severed almonds (elective)

How to Prepare: Using parchment paper, line baking sheets and warm up the oven to 350 deg.F (175 deg.C). Blend the oats, shredded coconut, almond flour, baking soda, ginger, and salt in a big basin. Mix until everything is well distributed. To ensure that the melted coconut oil, maple syrup, egg, and vanilla essence are thoroughly mixed together, put them in a distinct bowl and whisk them together. While mixing constantly, carefully incorporate the wet components into the dry components until a dough is formed. The grated carrot and Severed almonds, if using, should be folded in and combined. The dough should be dropped onto the baking sheets that have been prepared, with a distance of approximately 2 inches between each tbsp. For 12 to 15 minutes, or until the edges are a golden brown color, bake the cakes. The cookies should be allowed to cool for a couple of minutes on the baking sheets before being transferred to wire racks to finish cooling and becoming absolutely cool.

Nutritional Info: Calories: 145 kcal, Carb: 16g, Protein: 3g, Fat: 9g, Fiber: 3g, Sugars: 7g

13. Frozen Strawberry-Chocolate Greek Yogurt

Packed with protein and probiotics, this is an excellent option for men over 60, especially those following intermittent fasting. The high protein content helps maintain muscle mass, while probiotics support gut health. Plus, the natural sugars from honey and strawberries provide a satisfying energy boost during your eating window.

(Prep Time: 10 minutes | Freeze Time: 180 minutes | Servings: 32)

Ingredients:

- 1 cup sliced strawberries
- 2 tbsp honey
- ¼ cup chocolate chips
- 3 cups plain Greek yogurt
- 1 tsp vanilla extract

Instructions: Cover a baking sheet with parchment paper. In a medium mixing bowl, blend the Greek yogurt, honey, and vanilla extract. Spread the yogurt mixture on the lined baking sheet, forming a rectangle. Sprinkle the chocolate chips over the yogurt and arrange the sliced strawberries on top. The baking sheet should be placed in the freezer and left there for almost 3 hours, or until the yoghurt has reached a very solid consistency. The yoghurt should be cut into pieces and served once it has been frozen.

Nutritional Info: Fat: 1.3g; Protein: 2g; Sodium: 7.6mg

14. Frozen Peach-Mint Greek Yogurt Bites

This dish offers a refreshing and nutrient-packed snack option for men over 60 practicing intermittent fasting. The protein-rich Greek yogurt and healthy fats from pistachios support muscle maintenance, while the peaches provide a dose of antioxidants. Mint and lime include a refreshing twist, making these bites perfect for a light, energizing treat during your fasting breaks.

(Servings: 12 | Prep Time: 10 minutes | Freeze Time: 180 minutes)

Ingredients:

- 1/3 cup fresh peach slices (or canned peaches in natural juice, drained)
- 2 tsps agave syrup
- 1 tbsp severed pistachios
- 1 cup plain Greek yogurt
- 1/3 tsp mint extract (or finely severed fresh mint)
- 1/3 tsp lime zest

Instructions: Prepare a rectangular baking sheet or tray by covering it with parchment paper. Greek yoghurt, agave syrup, mint extract, and lime zest should be mixed together in a basin of medium size until thoroughly blended. The mixture should be thoroughly mixed and smooth. Make a rectangle with a thickness of approximately a quarter of an inch by spreading the yoghurt mixture onto the baking sheet that has been prepared. On top of the yoghurt, sprinkle the severed pistachios in a uniform manner, and then put the peach slices in a decorative pattern. Take the baking sheet and put it in the freezer.

Allow it to freeze for almost 3 hours, or until the yoghurt has reached the desired consistency. Once the yoghurt has been frozen, split it up or chop it into bite-sized pieces, and present it as soon as possible. Freeze any leftovers in a container that is airtight and store them in the freezer.

Nutritional Info: Calories: 35kcal | Fat: 1g | Carb: 4g | Sugar: 3g | Protein: 2g

---

15. Cucumber Mint Raspberry Sorbet

For men over 60 following intermittent fasting, this sorbet offers a low-calorie, hydrating treat that supports digestive health. The natural sugars from the fruit provide a gentle energy boost after a fasting window, while cucumber and mint aid in reducing inflammation and promoting a calm digestive system.

(Persons: 2 | Ready in: 15 minutes | Freezing Time: 4-6 hours)

Necessary Items:

- Fresh cucumber juice (from 1/2 big cucumber): 1/3 cup
- Fresh raspberry puree (from 3/4 cup raspberries): 1/4 cup
- Water: 1/3 cup
- Agave syrup or honey: 2 tbsps
- Fresh mint leaves, finely severed: 1 tbsp
- Lemon juice: 1 tbsp
- Fresh mint leaves for garnish (elective)

How to Prepare: In a small saucepan, blend the water and agave syrup (or honey). Heat at middling temp., stirring until dissolved to create a light syrup. Let the syrup cool to room temp. Once cooled, mix the syrup with the fresh cucumber juice, raspberry puree, and lemon juice. Stir well to blend the flavors. After pouring the liquid into an ice cream maker, churn it according to the instructions that were supplied by the manufacturer throughout the manufacturing process. The sorbet should be brought to a smooth and creamy consistency after roughly 20 to 25 minutes, or until it reaches that point. Just before finishing the churning process, include the finely severed mint leaves to infuse the sorbet with a refreshing hint of mint. Transfer the sorbet to a sealed container and freeze for 4-6 hours until firm. Present the Cucumber Mint Raspberry Sorbet in chilled bowls or glasses, garnishing with fresh mint leaves if desired.

Nutritional Info: Cal: 120kcal, Carb: 32g, Sugars: 29g, Protein: 1g Fiber: 2g

---

16. Almond Butter and Apple Sushi Rolls

Ideal for an energy boost during or after intermittent fasting, this simple dish offers high fiber, healthy fats, and a balance of natural sugars. For men over 60 practicing intermittent fasting, this snack is easy on digestion and packed with nutrients that support heart health, blood sugar balance, and energy levels. Almonds provide plant-based protein and magnesium, while apples and whole grains deliver fiber for gut health.

(Persons: 2 | Ready in: 10 minutes)

Necessary Items:

- Large whole-wheat tortillas: 2
- Ripe apples (finely cut): 2

- Almond butter (or sunflower seed butter): 4 tbsps
- Maple syrup: 2 tbsps
- Severed walnuts: 1/4 cup
- Ground nutmeg: 1/4 tsp
- Fresh berries (elective) for garnish

How to Prepare. Put the whole-wheat tortillas on a clean surface. Warm the almond butter in a microwave-safe bowl for about 20 seconds, making it easier to spread. Spread the warmed almond butter evenly over each tortilla. Drizzle 1 tbsp of maple syrup over each tortilla. Arrange the finely cut apples on the edge of each tortilla, layering them carefully. Sprinkle 2 tbsps of severed walnuts over the apples. Include a dash of ground nutmeg for a warm, spiced flavor. Roll up the tortillas tightly, starting from the edge with the apple slices, tucking in the sides as you go to create a sushi-like roll. Using a knife that is sharp, cut each roll into pieces that are suitable for nibbling. Optional: Garnish with fresh berries for extra color.

Info: Cal: 350 kcal, Carb: 60g, Sugars: 28g, Protein: 8g, Fat: 10g, Sodium: 250mg, Fiber: 7g

17. Nutty Oat Energy Bites

These bites provide a delightful blend of nutty flavors with the added benefit of flaxseeds, offering a boost of omega-3 fatty acids, which are crucial for heart health. For men over 60 practicing intermittent fasting, these bites offer an excellent source of energy during eating windows. The combination of cashews, oats, and dates supports heart health, while peanut butter adds plant-based protein to help maintain muscle mass during fasting periods.

(Persons: 12-15 energy balls | Ready in: 15 minutes)

Necessary Items:

- Cashews: 1 cup
- Medjool dates, pitted: 1 cup
- Rolled oats: 1/4 cup
- Peanut butter (or any nut butter): 2 tbsps
- Flaxseeds, ground: 1 tbsp
- Vanilla extract: 1 tsp
- Ground nutmeg: 1/4 tsp
- Sea salt: A pinch
- Water (if needed): 1-2 tbsps
- Optional: Crushed cashews or flaxseeds for rolling

How to Prepare. In a food processor, pulse the cashews until finely severed. Include the pitted dates, rolled oats, peanut butter, ground flaxseeds, vanilla extract, nutmeg, and sea salt. Blend until the mixture forms a sticky dough. If it appears too dry, include 1-2 tbsps of water and pulse again until combined. Stop occasionally to scrape down the sides for even mixing. Roll the dough into small balls, about 1 to 1.5 inches in diameter. Optional: Roll the energy bites in crushed cashews or ground flaxseeds for added texture. Put on a pan that has been covered with parchment paper and put it in the fridge for almost half an hour to allow it to set. You may keep it in the fridge for almost two weeks if you store it in a sealed container.

Nutritional Info: Calories: 135 kcal, Carbohydrates: 15g, Sugars: 10g, Protein: 3g, Fat: 7g, Sodium: 1mg, Fiber: 3g

18. Mixed Berry Yogurt Parfait

This parfait is an ideal choice for men over 60 adhering to intermittent fasting. The Greek yogurt provides a rich source of protein, essential for muscle maintenance and overall health. Berries are packed with antioxidants, which support heart health and cognitive function. The granola adds fiber and energy to sustain you through fasting periods. The inclusion of honey or maple syrup allows you to adjust sweetness without compromising nutritional balance.

(Persons: 2 | Ready in: 10 minutes)

Necessary Items:

- Greek yogurt (plain or vanilla flavored): 1 cup
- Mixed berries (strawberries, blueberries, raspberries, or your choice): 1 cup
- Granola: 1/2 cup
- Honey or maple syrup (elective for added sweetness): 2 tbsps
- Fresh mint leaves for garnish (elective)

How to Prepare. Wash and prepare the mixed berries. If using strawberries, remove the stems and slice them. In the event that you would like a layer of yogurt that is sweeter, blend the Greek yogurt with honey or maple syrup in a bowl. Adapt the level of sweetness to your preferences. Take two serving glasses or bowls. Start by layering the bottom of each glass with a spoonful of Greek yogurt. A layer of mixed berries should be placed on top of the yoghurt dish. A layer of granola should be sprinkled on top of the berries. It is possible to make your own granola or purchase it from a store. Repeat the layers - yogurt, berries, and granola - until the glasses are filled. Finish with a dollop of yogurt on the top layer and garnish with a few fresh berries and mint leaves if desired. Present instantly or refrigerate until ready to eat.

Nutritional Info: Calories: 250 kcal, Carbohydrates: 43g, Sugars: 19g, Protein: 13g, Fat: 4g, Fiber: 6g, Calcium: 150mg, Vitamin C: 35mg

90-Day Intermittent Fasting Meal Plan for Men Over 60
16:8 (16 hours fasting, 8 hours eating)

> ➤ **Fasting Period:** 8:00 PM to 12:00 PM
> ➤ **Eating Window:** 12:00 PM to 8:00 PM

The 16:8 intermittent fasting method, involving a 16-hour fasting period and an 8-hour eating window, is particularly well-suited for men over 60. This approach offers a balanced way to manage fasting and eating, aligning with the natural eating rhythms of many older adults. It provides the opportunity to enjoy three nutritious meals within the designated eating period. The 90-day meal plan outlined here supports men in their intermittent fasting journey, featuring a range of nutrient-rich breakfast, lunch, dinner, snack, and dessert options. Each meal is thoughtfully designed to deliver essential vitamins and minerals, promoting overall health and vitality. With a focus on balanced proteins, healthy fats, and carbohydrates, the plan meets the specific dietary needs of men over 60, enhancing both satisfaction and energy levels throughout the day.

Day 1

Breakfast: Power Protein Smoothie

Lunch: Lemon Herb Salmon with Roasted Brussels Sprouts

Dinner: Honey Sesame Salmon

Snack/Dessert: Almond Butter Cookies

Day 2

Breakfast: High-Protein Pancakes

Lunch: Grilled Eggplant and Spinach Panini

Dinner: Honey Garlic Tofu

Snack/Dessert: Berry Chia Seed Smoothie

Day 3

Breakfast: Egg and Avocado on Sweet Potato Toast with Sautéed Kale

Lunch: Sweet Potato and Black Bean Burrito

Dinner: Pork Tenderloin Stuffed with Apple, Walnuts, and Sage

Day 46

Breakfast: Egg and Cheese Quesadilla

Lunch: Lemon Herb Chicken and Veggie Skewers

Dinner: Citrus-Dijon Salmon with Roasted Cauliflower and Carrots

Snack/Dessert: Frozen Strawberry-Chocolate Greek Yogurt

Day 47

Breakfast: Banana Walnut Oatmeal

Lunch: Cauliflower Noodle Casserole

Dinner: Coconut Curried Pumpkin Soup

Snack/Dessert: Peanut Butter Oatmeal Chocolate Chip Cookies

Day 48

Breakfast: Prune Walnut Energy Bites

Lunch: Grilled Eggplant and Spinach Panini

Dinner: Grilled Lemon Garlic Chicken Breasts

Snack/Dessert: Baked Pears with

Snack/Dessert: Chocolate Avocado Pudding

Cinnamon and Pecans

Day 4

Breakfast: Sweet Potato and Turkey Breakfast Burritos

Lunch: Lemon Herb Chicken and Veggie Skewers

Dinner: Roasted Carrots with Garlic and Herb Infusion

Snack/Dessert: Spiced Almond-Coconut Energy Bites

Day 49

Breakfast: Quinoa Breakfast Bowl with Apple and Walnuts

Lunch: Chicken Salad with Walnuts and Grapes

Dinner: Maple-Balsamic Glazed Chicken Thighs with Roasted Butternut Squash

Snack/Dessert: Frozen Peach-Mint Greek Yogurt Bites

Day 5

Breakfast: High-Fiber Banana Nut Porridge

Lunch: Lemon Basil Grilled Cod

Dinner: Herb-Crusted Baked Haddock

Snack/Dessert: Frozen Strawberry-Chocolate Greek Yogurt

Day 50

Breakfast: Blueberry Spinach Smoothie

Lunch: Butternut Squash and Spinach Risotto

Dinner: Pork Tenderloin Stuffed with Apple, Walnuts, and Sage

Snack/Dessert: Chocolate Avocado Pudding

Day 6

Breakfast: Honey Almond Quinoa Granola

Lunch: Butternut Squash and Spinach Risotto

Dinner: Maple-Balsamic Glazed Chicken Thighs with Roasted Butternut Squash

Snack/Dessert: Creamy Coconut Rice Pudding with Chia Seeds

Day 51

Breakfast: Apple Cinnamon Almond Scones

Lunch: Mediterranean Shrimp Salad with Lemon Tahini Dressing

Dinner: Honey Sesame Salmon

Snack/Dessert: Spiced Almond-Coconut Energy Bites

Day 7

Breakfast: Savory Lentil & Veggie Scramble

Lunch: Chickpea and Carrot Stew with Couscous

Dinner: Citrus-Dijon Salmon with Roasted Cauliflower and Carrots

Snack/Dessert: Almond Butter and Apple Sushi Rolls

Day 52

Breakfast: Egg Scramble with Sweet Potatoes

Lunch: Lemon Basil Grilled Cod

Dinner: Grilled Lamb Chops with Basil Pesto and Roasted Sweet Potatoes

Snack/Dessert: Frozen Strawberry-Chocolate Greek Yogurt

Day 8

Breakfast: Apple Cinnamon Almond Scones

Lunch: Chicken Salad with Walnuts and Grapes

Dinner: Grilled Lemon Garlic Chicken Breasts

Snack/Dessert: Mixed Berry Yogurt Parfait

Day 9

Breakfast: Banana Walnut Oatmeal

Lunch: Cauliflower Noodle Casserole

Dinner: Ricotta and Sun-Dried Tomato Stuffed Salmon

Snack/Dessert: Nutty Oat Energy Bites

Day 10

Breakfast: Blueberry Almond Muffins

Lunch: Mediterranean Shrimp Salad with Lemon Tahini Dressing

Dinner: Sweet Potato and Rosemary Risotto

Snack/Dessert: Avocado-Cocoa Mousse with a Hint of Mint

Day 11

Breakfast: Egg Scramble with Sweet Potatoes

Lunch: Zucchini Noodles with Spicy Peanut Sauce

Dinner: Lemon Rosemary Grilled Swordfish

Snack/Dessert: Baked Pears with Cinnamon and Pecans

Day 12

Breakfast: Sunflower Seed Butter Apple Toast

Lunch: Greek-Style Chicken Salad Bowl

Dinner: Grilled Lamb Chops with Basil

Day 53

Breakfast: Sunflower Seed Butter Apple Toast

Lunch: Lemon Herb Chicken and Veggie Skewers

Dinner: Honey Garlic Tofu

Snack/Dessert: Coconut Chia Pudding with Mango

Day 54

Breakfast: Cottage Cheese and Veggie Lettuce Wraps

Lunch: Greek-Style Chicken Salad Bowl

Dinner: Citrus-Dijon Salmon with Roasted Cauliflower and Carrots

Snack/Dessert: Avocado-Cocoa Mousse with a Hint of Mint

Day 55

Breakfast: Savory Lentil & Veggie Scramble

Lunch: Zucchini Noodles with Spicy Peanut Sauce

Dinner: Grilled Lemon Garlic Chicken Breasts

Snack/Dessert: Peanut Butter Oatmeal Chocolate Chip Cookies

Day 56

Breakfast: High-Protein Pancakes

Lunch: Roasted Cauliflower and Broccoli Gratin

Dinner: Walnut-Crusted Turkey Cutlets

Snack/Dessert: Mixed Berry Yogurt Parfait

Day 57

Breakfast: Honey Almond Quinoa Granola

Lunch: Avocado and Kale Soup

Dinner: Stuffed Zucchini with Quinoa

Pesto and Roasted Sweet Potatoes

Snack/Dessert: Herbed Almonds with Rosemary

Day 13

Breakfast: Egg and Cheese Quesadilla

Lunch: Bell Peppers Stuffed with Quinoa, Spinach, and Feta

Dinner: Eggplant Parmesan with Spinach and Avocado Salad

Snack/Dessert: Carrot Oatmeal Raisin Muffins

Day 14

Breakfast: Prune Walnut Energy Bites

Lunch: Caper and Bean Salad with Tuna

Dinner: Walnut-Crusted Turkey Cutlets

Snack/Dessert: Coconut Chia Pudding with Mango

Day 15

Breakfast: Chickpea and Carrot Spread Sandwich

Lunch: Avocado and Kale Soup

Dinner: Ginger-Lime Chicken with Cucumber and Bell Pepper Salad

Snack/Dessert: Spiced Almond-Coconut Energy Bites

Day 16

Breakfast: Cottage Cheese and Veggie Lettuce Wraps

Lunch: Tropical Mango and Chicken Lettuce Wraps

Dinner: Stuffed Zucchini with Quinoa and Turkey

Snack/Dessert: Herbed Almonds with Rosemary

Day 17

Breakfast: Greek Yogurt with Apple and Almonds

and Turkey

Snack/Dessert: Herbed Almonds with Rosemary

Day 58

Breakfast: Honey Almond Quinoa Granola

Lunch: Avocado and Kale Soup

Dinner: Stuffed Zucchini with Quinoa and Turkey

Snack/Dessert: Herbed Almonds with Rosemary

Day 59

Breakfast: Quinoa Breakfast Bowl with Apple and Walnuts

Lunch: Chickpea and Carrot Stew with Couscous

Dinner: Pork Tenderloin Stuffed with Apple, Walnuts, and Sage

Snack/Dessert: Frozen Peach-Mint Greek Yogurt Bites

Day 60

Breakfast: Blueberry Almond Muffins

Lunch: Cauliflower Noodle Casserole

Dinner: Honey Sesame Salmon

Snack/Dessert: Avocado-Cocoa Mousse with a Hint of Mint

Day 61

Breakfast: Prune Walnut Energy Bites

Lunch: Grilled Eggplant and Spinach Panini

Dinner: Coconut Curried Pumpkin Soup

Snack/Dessert: Frozen Strawberry-Chocolate Greek Yogurt

Day 62

Breakfast: Egg Scramble with Sweet Potatoes

Lunch: Spinach and Goat Cheese Omelette

Dinner: Citrus-Basil Baked Cod with Roasted Cherry Tomatoes

Snack/Dessert: Avocado-Cocoa Mousse with a Hint of Mint

Day 18

Breakfast: Blueberry Spinach Smoothie

Lunch: Roasted Cauliflower and Broccoli Gratin

Dinner: Maple-Balsamic Glazed Chicken Thighs with Roasted Butternut Squash

Snack/Dessert: Almond Butter Cookies

Day 19

Breakfast: Quinoa Breakfast Bowl with Apple and Walnuts

Lunch: Lemon Garlic Shrimp Sauté

Dinner: Roasted Carrots with Garlic and Herb Infusion
Snack/Dessert: Frozen Peach-Mint Greek Yogurt Bites

Day 20

Breakfast: Baked Pears with Almonds and Cinnamon

Lunch: Butternut Squash and Spinach Risotto

Dinner: Grilled Lemon Garlic Chicken Breasts

Snack/Dessert: Nutty Oat Energy Bites

Day 21

Breakfast: Power Protein Smoothie

Lunch: Sweet Potato and Black Bean Burrito

Dinner: Herb-Crusted Baked Haddock

Lunch: Lemon Herb Chicken and Veggie Skewers

Dinner: Grilled Lemon Garlic Chicken Breasts

Snack/Dessert: Peanut Butter Oatmeal Chocolate Chip Cookies

Day 63

Breakfast: High-Fiber Banana Nut Porridge

Lunch: Zucchini Noodles with Spicy Peanut Sauce

Dinner: Citrus-Basil Baked Cod with Roasted Cherry Tomatoes

Snack/Dessert: Coconut Chia Pudding with Mango

Day 64

Breakfast: Egg and Avocado on Sweet Potato Toast with Sautéed Kale

Lunch: Sweet Potato and Black Bean Burrito

Dinner: Grilled Lamb Chops with Basil Pesto and Roasted Sweet Potatoes

Snack/Dessert: Baked Pears with Cinnamon and Pecans

Day 65

Breakfast: Cottage Cheese and Veggie Lettuce Wraps

Lunch: Chicken Salad with Walnuts and Grapes

Dinner: Maple-Balsamic Glazed Chicken Thighs with Roasted Butternut Squash

Snack/Dessert: Frozen Peach-Mint Greek Yogurt Bites

Day 66

Breakfast: Sunflower Seed Butter Apple Toast

Lunch: Spinach and Goat Cheese Omelette

Dinner: Citrus-Dijon Salmon with

Snack/Dessert: Chocolate Avocado Pudding

Roasted Cauliflower and Carrots

Snack/Dessert: Mixed Berry Yogurt Parfait

Day 22

Breakfast: High-Protein Pancakes

Lunch: Lemon Herb Chicken and Veggie Skewers

Dinner: Ricotta and Sun-Dried Tomato Stuffed Salmon

Snack/Dessert: Mixed Berry Yogurt Parfait

Day 23

Breakfast: Egg and Avocado on Sweet Potato Toast with Sautéed Kale

Lunch: Mediterranean Shrimp Salad with Lemon Tahini Dressing

Dinner: Lemon Rosemary Grilled Swordfish

Snack/Dessert: Carrot Oatmeal Raisin Muffins

Day 24

Breakfast: Sweet Potato and Turkey Breakfast Burritos

Lunch: Greek-Style Chicken Salad Bowl

Dinner: Grilled Lamb Chops with Basil Pesto and Roasted Sweet Potatoes

Snack/Dessert: Spiced Almond-Coconut Energy Bites

Day 25

Breakfast: High-Fiber Banana Nut Porridge

Lunch: Cauliflower Noodle Casserole

Dinner: Citrus-Dijon Salmon with Roasted Cauliflower and Carrots

Snack/Dessert: Almond Butter and Apple Sushi Rolls

Day 26

Breakfast: Honey Almond Quinoa Granola

Day 67

Breakfast: Power Protein Smoothie

Lunch: Mediterranean Shrimp Salad with Lemon Tahini Dressing

Dinner: Pork Tenderloin Stuffed with Apple, Walnuts, and Sage

Snack/Dessert: Chocolate Avocado Pudding

Day 68

Breakfast: Apple Cinnamon Almond Scones

Lunch: Greek-Style Chicken Salad Bowl

Dinner: Herb-Crusted Baked Haddock

Snack/Dessert: Peanut Butter Oatmeal Chocolate Chip Cookies

Day 69

Breakfast: Blueberry Spinach Smoothie

Lunch: Roasted Cauliflower and Broccoli Gratin

Dinner: Honey Garlic Tofu

Snack/Dessert: Spiced Almond-Coconut Energy Bites

Day 70

Breakfast: Honey Almond Quinoa Granola

Lunch: Butternut Squash and Spinach Risotto

Dinner: Grilled Lemon Garlic Chicken Breasts

Snack/Dessert: Herbed Almonds with Rosemary

Day 71

Breakfast: Egg Scramble with Sweet Potatoes

Lunch: Sweet Potato and Black Bean Burrito

Dinner: Grilled Lemon Garlic Chicken Breasts

Snack/Dessert: Herbed Almonds with Rosemary

Day 27

Breakfast: Savory Lentil & Veggie Scramble

Lunch: Lemon Basil Grilled Cod

Dinner: Eggplant Parmesan with Spinach and Avocado Salad

Snack/Dessert: Creamy Coconut Rice Pudding with Chia Seeds

Day 28

Breakfast: Apple Cinnamon Almond Scones

Lunch: Bell Peppers Stuffed with Quinoa, Spinach, and Feta

Dinner: Honey Sesame Salmon

Snack/Dessert: Avocado-Cocoa Mousse with a Hint of Mint

Day 29

Breakfast: Banana Walnut Oatmeal

Lunch: Chickpea and Carrot Stew with Couscous

Dinner: Maple-Balsamic Glazed Chicken Thighs with Roasted Butternut Squash

Snack/Dessert: Baked Pears with Cinnamon and Pecans

Day 30

Breakfast: Blueberry Almond Muffins

Lunch: Avocado and Kale Soup

Dinner: Grilled Lemon Garlic Chicken Breasts

Snack/Dessert: Nutty Oat Energy Bites

Lunch: Zucchini Noodles with Spicy Peanut Sauce

Dinner: Citrus-Basil Baked Cod with Roasted Cherry Tomatoes

Snack/Dessert: Avocado-Cocoa Mousse with a Hint of Mint

Day 72

Breakfast: Cottage Cheese and Veggie Lettuce Wraps

Lunch: Chickpea and Carrot Stew with Couscous

Dinner: Grilled Lamb Chops with Basil Pesto and Roasted Sweet Potatoes

Snack/Dessert: Frozen Strawberry-Chocolate Greek Yogurt

Day 73

Breakfast: Quinoa Breakfast Bowl with Apple and Walnuts

Lunch: Cauliflower Noodle Casserole

Dinner: Ricotta and Sun-Dried Tomato Stuffed Salmon

Snack/Dessert: Mixed Berry Yogurt Parfait

Day 74

Breakfast: Banana Walnut Oatmeal

Lunch: Lemon Herb Chicken and Veggie Skewers

Dinner: Pork Tenderloin Stuffed with Apple, Walnuts, and Sage

Snack/Dessert: Nutty Oat Energy Bites

Day 75

Breakfast: Blueberry Almond Muffins

Lunch: Sweet Potato and Black Bean Burrito

Dinner: Maple-Balsamic Glazed Chicken Thighs with Roasted Butternut Squash

Snack/Dessert: Coconut Chia Pudding

Day 31

Breakfast: Egg Scramble with Sweet Potatoes

Lunch: Spinach and Goat Cheese Omelette

Dinner: Herb-Crusted Baked Haddock

Snack/Dessert: Frozen Strawberry-Chocolate Greek Yogurt

Day 32

Breakfast: Sunflower Seed Butter Apple Toast

Lunch: Caper and Bean Salad with Tuna

Dinner: Pork Tenderloin Stuffed with Apple, Walnuts, and Sage

Snack/Dessert: Almond Butter Cookies

Day 33

Breakfast: Egg and Cheese Quesadilla

Lunch: Tropical Mango and Chicken Lettuce Wraps

Dinner: Citrus-Basil Baked Cod with Roasted Cherry Tomatoes

Snack/Dessert: Berry Chia Seed Smoothie

Day 34

Breakfast: Prune Walnut Energy Bites

Lunch: Butternut Squash and Spinach Risotto

Dinner: Roasted Carrots with Garlic and Herb Infusion

Snack/Dessert: Frozen Peach-Mint Greek Yogurt Bites

Day 35

Breakfast: Chickpea and Carrot Spread Sandwich

Lunch: Lemon Herb Salmon with Roasted Brussels Sprouts

Dinner: Walnut-Crusted Turkey Cutlets

with Mango

Day 76

Breakfast: Power Protein Smoothie

Lunch: Spinach and Goat Cheese Omelette

Dinner: Citrus-Dijon Salmon with Roasted Cauliflower and Carrots

Snack/Dessert: Peanut Butter Oatmeal Chocolate Chip Cookies

Day 77

Breakfast: High-Fiber Banana Nut Porridge

Lunch: Grilled Eggplant and Spinach Panini

Dinner: Grilled Lemon Garlic Chicken Breasts

Snack/Dessert: Frozen Peach-Mint Greek Yogurt Bites

Day 78

Breakfast: Savory Lentil & Veggie Scramble

Lunch: Greek-Style Chicken Salad Bowl

Dinner: Coconut Curried Pumpkin Soup

Snack/Dessert: Chocolate Avocado Pudding

Day 79

Breakfast: Egg and Cheese Quesadilla

Lunch: Mediterranean Shrimp Salad with Lemon Tahini Dressing

Dinner: Herb-Crusted Baked Haddock

Snack/Dessert: Mixed Berry Yogurt Parfait

Day 80

Breakfast: Honey Almond Quinoa Granola

Lunch: Roasted Cauliflower and Broccoli Gratin

Dinner: Grilled Lamb Chops with Basil

Snack/Dessert: Coconut Carrot Crunch Cookies

Day 36

Breakfast: Quinoa Breakfast Bowl with Apple and Walnuts

Lunch: Lemon Herb Salmon with Roasted Brussels Sprouts

Dinner: Citrus-Basil Baked Cod with Roasted Cherry Tomatoes

Snack/Dessert: Peanut Butter Oatmeal Chocolate Chip Cookies

Day 37

Breakfast: Egg and Avocado on Sweet Potato Toast with Sautéed Kale

Lunch: Chickpea and Carrot Stew with Couscous

Dinner: Herb-Crusted Baked Haddock

Snack/Dessert: Coconut Chia Pudding with Mango

Day 38

Breakfast: High-Protein Pancakes

Lunch: Zucchini Noodles with Spicy Peanut Sauce

Dinner: Pork Tenderloin Stuffed with Apple, Walnuts, and Sage

Snack/Dessert: Frozen Strawberry-Chocolate Greek Yogurt

Day 39

Breakfast: Savory Lentil & Veggie Scramble

Lunch: Chicken Salad with Walnuts and Grapes

Dinner: Honey Garlic Tofu

Snack/Dessert: Spiced Almond-Coconut Energy Bites

Day 40

Breakfast: Honey Almond Quinoa Granola

Pesto and Roasted Sweet Potatoes

Snack/Dessert: Spiced Almond-Coconut Energy Bites

Day 81

Breakfast: Quinoa Breakfast Bowl with Apple and Walnuts

Lunch: Lemon Herb Salmon with Roasted Brussels Sprouts

Dinner: Ricotta and Sun-Dried Tomato Stuffed Salmon

Snack/Dessert: Herbed Almonds with Rosemary

Day 82

Breakfast: Sunflower Seed Butter Apple Toast

Lunch: Zucchini Noodles with Spicy Peanut Sauce

Dinner: Grilled Lemon Garlic Chicken Breasts

Snack/Dessert: Coconut Chia Pudding with Mango

Day 83

Breakfast: Cottage Cheese and Veggie Lettuce Wraps

Lunch: Chickpea and Carrot Stew with Couscous

Dinner: Honey Garlic Tofu

Snack/Dessert: Nutty Oat Energy Bites

Day 84

Breakfast: Power Protein Smoothie

Lunch: Spinach and Goat Cheese Omelette

Dinner: Grilled Lamb Chops with Basil Pesto and Roasted Sweet Potatoes

Snack/Dessert: Mixed Berry Yogurt Parfait

Day 85

Breakfast: Apple Cinnamon Almond Scones

Lunch: Mediterranean Shrimp Salad with Lemon Tahini Dressing

Dinner: Maple-Balsamic Glazed Chicken Thighs with Roasted Butternut Squash

Snack/Dessert: Avocado-Cocoa Mousse with a Hint of Mint

Day 41
Breakfast: Blueberry Almond Muffins

Lunch: Sweet Potato and Black Bean Burrito

Dinner: Grilled Lemon Garlic Chicken Breasts

Snack/Dessert: Frozen Peach-Mint Greek Yogurt Bites

Day 42
Breakfast: Cottage Cheese and Veggie Lettuce Wraps

Lunch: Spinach and Goat Cheese Omelette

Dinner: Herbed Chicken with Swiss Cheese

Snack/Dessert: Mixed Berry Yogurt Parfait

Day 43
Breakfast: Power Protein Smoothie

Lunch: Roasted Cauliflower and Broccoli Gratin

Dinner: Walnut-Crusted Turkey Cutlets

Snack/Dessert: Herbed Almonds with Rosemary

Day 44
Breakfast: Egg Scramble with Sweet Potatoes

Lunch: Avocado and Kale Soup

Dinner: Grilled Lamb Chops with Basil Pesto and Roasted Sweet Potatoes

Lunch: Sweet Potato and Black Bean Burrito

Dinner: Citrus-Dijon Salmon with Roasted Cauliflower and Carrots

Snack/Dessert: Chocolate Avocado Pudding

Day 86
Breakfast: High-Protein Pancakes

Lunch: Mediterranean Shrimp Salad with Lemon Tahini Dressing

Dinner: Maple-Balsamic Glazed Chicken Thighs with Roasted Butternut Squash

Snack/Dessert: Peanut Butter Oatmeal Chocolate Chip Cookies

Day 87
Breakfast: Banana Walnut Oatmeal

Lunch: Roasted Cauliflower and Broccoli Gratin

Dinner: Pork Tenderloin Stuffed with Apple, Walnuts, and Sage

Snack/Dessert: Frozen Peach-Mint Greek Yogurt Bites

Day 88
Breakfast: Savory Lentil & Veggie Scramble

Lunch: Grilled Eggplant and Spinach Panini

Dinner: Coconut Curried Pumpkin Soup

Snack/Dessert: Herbed Almonds with Rosemary

Day 89
Breakfast: Egg and Cheese Quesadilla

Lunch: Greek-Style Chicken Salad Bowl

Dinner: Herb-Crusted Baked Haddock

Snack/Dessert: Avocado-Cocoa Mousse with a Hint of Mint

Snack/Dessert: Coconut Chia Pudding with Mango

Day 45

Breakfast: High-Fiber Banana Nut Porridge

Lunch: Sweet Potato and Black Bean Quinoa Bowl

Dinner: Ricotta and Sun-Dried Tomato Stuffed Salmon

Snack/Dessert: Nutty Oat Energy Bites

Day 90

Breakfast: Cottage Cheese and Veggie Lettuce Wraps

Lunch: Spinach and Goat Cheese Omelette

Dinner: Grilled Lemon Garlic Chicken Breasts

Snack/Dessert: Frozen Strawberry-Chocolate Greek Yogurt

Congratulations On Completing The 90-Day Intermittent Fasting Meal Plan!

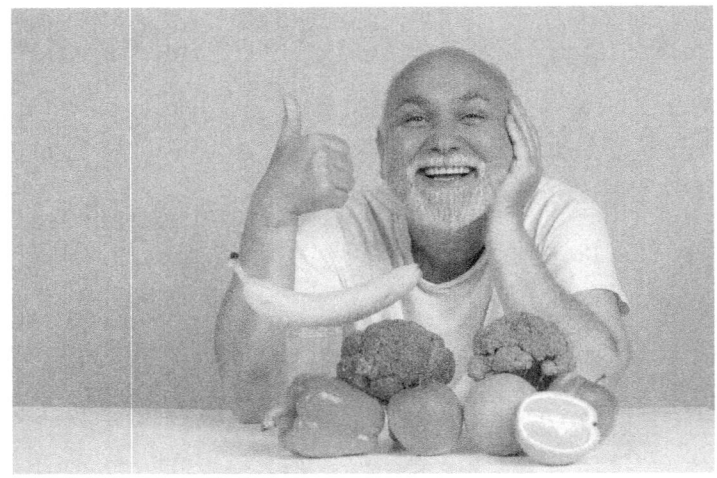

By now, you should have adapted to this eating pattern and experienced its potential benefits. Remember to continue making mindful food choices and listening to your body's needs.

Conclusion

This comprehensive guide has taken you on a journey crafted to address the specific needs and goals of men in their later years. Throughout these chapters, we've delved into the transformative potential of intermittent fasting, providing you with the insights, tools, and inspiration to confidently adopt this lifestyle. We began by exploring the principles of intermittent fasting, breaking down its core concepts, and highlighting the science behind its many health benefits. With a focus on men over 60, the fasting strategies presented here were tailored to meet your unique requirements, offering practical guidance on how to start and maintain this dietary approach safely and effectively. As we age, physiological changes naturally occur, and intermittent fasting can be a powerful tool to navigate these challenges, helping to improve your overall well-being. This book aimed to integrate fasting seamlessly into your life, encouraging you to build confidence and resilience as you progressed. We also explored nutrition, supplements, and additional resources to support your fasting journey, including the benefits of blending traditional medicine and natural remedies to enhance your results. Recognizing the importance of staying physically active, we underscored the powerful connection between intermittent fasting and exercise. We've provided a range of exercise plans suitable for men over 60, designed to promote overall wellness, strength, and vitality as you continue to age. Building a support network is key to long-term success, so we've offered advice on finding reliable resources, connecting with others who share similar goals, and involving those closest to you in your fasting routine. Surrounding yourself with a supportive community can make the journey not only easier but also more rewarding. No journey through intermittent fasting would be complete without nourishing, satisfying meals. The recipes included in this book were carefully chosen to support your fasting goals without sacrificing flavor or enjoyment. From balanced breakfasts to hearty lunches and dinners, and even delicious snacks and desserts, we've ensured that healthy eating can remain a pleasurable experience. Intermittent fasting isn't just about what you eat or when you eat—it's about transforming your lifestyle. It's a journey of renewal, strength, and self-discovery. We hope that the knowledge and strategies you've gained from this book have empowered you to take on this new chapter with confidence. Remember, age is simply a number. It's never too late to make changes that will improve your health and vitality. Celebrate the milestones you reach along the way, listen to your body, and continue to explore the vast potential of intermittent fasting. Each step forward brings you closer to a healthier, more energetic, and fulfilling life. As you continue this journey, know that the path might have its challenges, but the rewards of increased energy, improved health, and a renewed passion for life make it all worthwhile. The power to create a vibrant, healthy future lies in your hands—embrace it with optimism and purpose.

BONUS 1

BONUS ANTI-INFLAMMATORY RECIPES

Dear Reader,

We're thrilled to offer you our bonus "ANTI-INFLAMMATORY RECIPES"!

Simply send an email to **oliviastokes162@gmail.com**

with the subject line **BONUS ANTI-INFLAMMATORY RECIPES**, and you'll receive a PDF filled with quick and delicious recipes designed to help you reduce inflammation naturally and support your overall health.

BONUS 2

MUSIC FOR FASTING

Scan the QR code and listen to curated tunes

Dear Reader,

Thank you for taking the time to explore "Intermittent Fasting for Men Over 60." As the author, my goal is to inspire people to take control of their health through mindful eating and balanced nutrition.

our feedback is invaluable, both to me and to others who may be considering this book. By sharing your thoughts and experiences, you not only help me grow as an author but also assist fellow readers in making informed decisions about their own health journeys.

would greatly appreciate it if you could take a moment to leave a review on Amazon. Whether you found the recipes helpful, the information insightful, or have suggestions for improvement, your feedback is essential and deeply valued.

Leaving a review is simple. Just scan the QR code below with your smartphone, and you'll be taken directly to the Amazon review page. Your honest review can make a meaningful impact, and I am grateful for your support in spreading the message of wellness and vitality.

Thank you for being a part of this journey.

Warm regards,

Olivia Stokes

Printed in Great Britain
by Amazon

56376950R00073